Woman In The Woods

KATHLEEN FARMER

INDIANA CAMP SUPPLY BOOKS

Pittsboro, Indiana

WOMAN IN THE WOODS

Copyright© 1976 by Kathleen Farmer

Published by
Indiana Camp Supply Books, Inc.
405 Osborne, Pittsboro, IN 46167

Library of Congress in Publication Data

Farmer, Kathleen, 1946-
　　Woman in the Woods.

　　Bibliography: p.
　　Includes index.
　　1. Outdoor recreation for women. 2. Women--Health and hygiene.
　　I. Title.　(GV191.64.F37　1980)　796'.01'94　80-22021
ISBN 0-934802-08-4 (pbk.)

Library of Congress Catalog Card Number: 80-22021

Printed in the U.S.A.

To Charlie—
the sky of my world, the spark of my ideas, the
spring overflowing with encouragement and belief that keeps me on course

Contents

Acknowledgments

The concept of *Woman in the Woods* came from Charlie, who considered my experiences worth sharing with others. The independence that enabled me to move from Cincinnati to Wyoming resulted from my parents, who taught me to be original, bold, and nonconforming. Much of the practical advice and insights in this book is the product of twenty outdoorswomen who took the time to answer my questions and share their personal thoughts with readers. Several even contributed photos. The confidence that the woods will exist for our grandchildren and beyond results from the concern of today's outdoorspeople. Thank you.

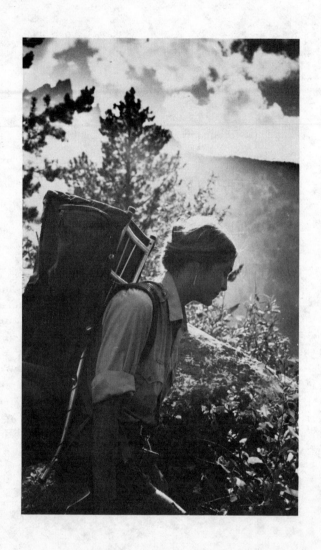

Introduction

You enjoy picnics, badminton, and the patio. You spend hours soaking up the summer sun; wish fall would never come, yet like to kick your way through the icing of the first snow. You have never considered yourself an outdoorsperson, but the fragrance of flowers, autumn colors, and the sound of a spring rain against the picture window hold special meaning to you.

You see, hear, and read a lot about backpacking, wilderness camping, and mountaineering and wonder how a person—especially a woman—can get involved in such activities. Where to begin is the question that arises repeatedly. How to broaden your outdoor experiences beyond the backyard, into the woods?

Woman in the Woods tells you everything you need to know to get along in the backwoods. How to stay clean and comfortable. How to feel feminine away from civilized conveniences. How to gain confidence. How to venture into the woods alone, yet secure. The basics of outdoor living, camping, rock hunting, fishing, and hunting are explained in a special way so they mean something to you.

Find out for yourself what to expect and how to prepare yourself for the adventure that is waiting for you in nature.

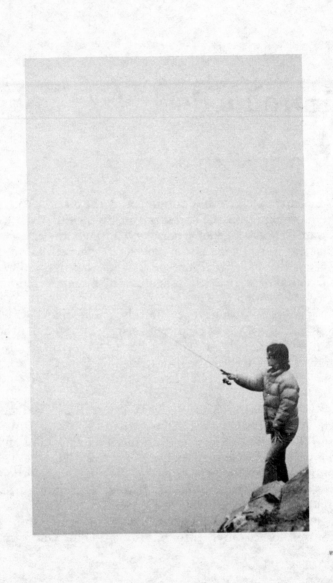

1

Learning About Nature Right Around Home

Imagine for a moment. A laughing, rushing stream, dancing over moss-speckled granite rocks, filling the gloom of dense Douglas fir and lodgepole pines with lightness and song. Look into the virgin water. There you are! Reflected. Part of the liquid motion, the basic vitality of nature. Bubbles shoot up, gently dimple your face, and lazily roll down your cheeks like tears of joy. Smell the damp pine and feel it sink into your mood and bones. You are there and nature is you.

Cross the embryonic river. Skip from one stone to another. Your hiking boots grip sure and secure. The opposite shore is uninterrupted by trails. Truly untamed, unexplored. Unhook the metal cup from your belt loop. Scoop up a mouthful of water. Transparent. Take a gulp. The cold fluid tingles tongue, gums, and teeth and transmits chills down the esophagus into the stomach. The wilds has entered you. Satisfying thirst, water is the first tie to this strangely inviting sphere. How to live freely, grow organically, recreate without TV, a car, and other mechanical devices. That is *woodswomanship*.

Ahead, a loud, unfamiliar call cracks the dawn. Through the silent trees it resounds, enlarging as it travels. What creature produces such a bold, demanding croak? "Be alert; be ready," it seems to warn. A huge black form circles high above the pines. Lodgepole trunks point skyward towards the raven, identifying him as the villain with the alarming voice. A scavenger, he lives off others. Consequently, he feels immortal. His time will never come.

Step gingerly on the ground blanketed with pine needles. You are walking on history. The earth's past. Right now the lodgpole pines and aspens are preparing the soil for spruce and fir trees. The immense size and overpopulation of the lodgepoles create shade. But their own seeds and shoots cannot survive without enough sunlight. Years pass and a young forest of spruce and fir replaces the lodgepole and aspen. The plant world is a continuous cycle. One population creates conditions suitable for the next community of plants. In the process, however, the original population's existence is threatened. It takes time—a hundred, maybe a thousand years.

Compared to civilization, nature operates in slow motion. The woodswoman likewise gears down to a less frantic pace. She takes time to see and sense the breadth of what appears on the surface to be so simple.

The thick woods gives way to a soft meadow, full of high grass, weeds, and golden willow bushes. Here the stream is dammed. Mud and willow and aspen branches are weaved expertly to produce a sturdy water blockade. A tepee made of twigs sits in the middle of the pond. The same architect—the beaver—designed both the dam and the lodge. Sit on a fallen log. Wait and watch.

Suddenly a muskrat with furry brown head, whiskers, and two tiny pointed ears appears on the surface. He swims to shore. The muskrat's senses scour the surroundings cautiously for signs of potential danger. Having poor eyesight, the muskrat relies on hearing, smell, and intuition to identify perils, such as hawks, coyotes, and mink. A fur-bearer, he is small compared to the beaver and has a long, thin, hairless tail. He sits on the grassy bank and munches.

A mallard duck splashes a loud landing. The muskrat

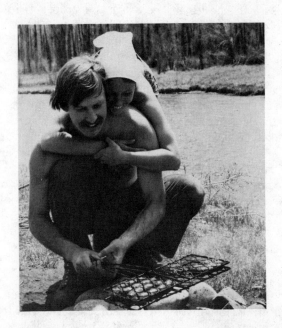

Nature gears you down, gives you time to appreciate the simple things.

quickly dives in, swims underwater towards the duck. The drake, his green head iridescent in the sunlight, anticipates the muskrat's antics. His loud-orange feet churn, propel him over the water surface, out of reach of the muskrat.

A grayish blue bird, built mostly of wings and legs, glides low over the willows like a prehistoric spirit. A great blue heron. He lands at the water's edge and stands statuelike. The neck curls close to the body, like a spring wound for action. The bill stabs the surface. It emerges with a squirming four-inch minnow. The heron stretches his neck and swallows. Wading three feet away, he spears another.

Peace. The beaver is the perfect host. He builds a dam to create a pond. It attracts a crowd of visitors: fish, birds, coyotes, moose, deer, muskrats, mink. Even anglers, photographers, and wildlife observers. The beaver gnaws down trees with his rust-colored chisellike teeth. In the pond he stores the trunks and branches. When a layer of ice seals off the pond, the beaver has a supply of food available near the underwater exit of his lodge.

Alongside the beaver pond, the sportswoman is just another living organism. She belongs to the human species—a female human. The alleged superiority of man is erased in the woods. With meager instinctive drives, a human is more vulnerable than other animals. An outdoorsperson relies on knowledge gained from others as well as from experience and inborn common sense. The "babe in the woods" is the ignorant human trying to apply city ways to nature.

Woodswomanship is confidence that you can cope with the elements. You believe in yourself and your ability to solve whatever situation arises in the outdoors. A never-ending process of self-education. No one knows everything about the wilds. But each trip teaches something.

The woman in the woods can be you.

Begin with yourself. Outdoor lore can be learned in the classroom. But putting the knowledge into practice takes gumption. Achieving self-confidence in the outdoors is a state of mind. It is based in a belief in yourself and a desire to discover what is happening outside the walls of your home. Concern and curiosity keep you going.

You cannot expect to go out in the wilds and immediately feel confident. Begin slowly. Experience nature step by step. Start with a seed of interest in the outdoors and watch it blossom into a flower of self-confidence and knowledge of nature and her ways.

WHERE TO GET INSTRUCTION IN OUTDOOR SPORTS

Several important aspects of woodswomanship can be understood only through personal experience. However, many outdoor activities can be learned faster, and more completely and safely from an instructor. Training eliminates trial and error. The student profits from the teacher's experience. Sports such as canoeing, scuba diving, skiing, and fly-fishing require initial training. Running a river or swishing down a slope can be the height of physical sensation or a terrifying, death-defying horror, depending on the level of instruction.

In addition, learning an outdoor sport gives a person direction. You will not be walking aimlessly on a trail trying to "communicate with nature." A sport helps bridge the gap between you and nature. Fishing, for example, directs interest outwards towards wild streams, unfathomable lakes. It is the excuse for getting outdoors often. While fishing, you expose yourself to nature and strengthen the common bond without realizing it.

Within your community, there are numerous opportunities to learn about nature. Local chapters of the YWCA, the Jewish Community Center, the American Red Cross, and the Coast Guard Auxiliary sponsor short (four to six weeks) training sessions. The Coast Guard Auxiliary teaches first-rate courses in navigation, sailing, boat handling, safety, and mechanics. The American Red Cross provides swimming and life-saving lessons. In some areas, they teach canoeing and scuba diving as well. The YWCA and the Jewish Community Center organize group skiing lessons, snowshoe trips, and physical fitness programs. The city newspaper advertises these classes. The local office of each of these agencies can give specifics of when, where, and how much.

Junior colleges, city colleges, and night schools offer courses on outdoor subjects in the adult education curriculum. Instruction in conservation, ecology, animal biology, forestry, and fish and game management is available. Popular local outdoor sports are usually the ones taught at the schools. Each section of the country features dominant outdoor activities. The Rocky Mountain states, for instance, are known for prime trout fishing and splendid downhill skiing. Missouri and Arkansas mean slow lazy rivers and sassy bass. Coastal and riverside cities focus on water-oriented sports—boating, water-skiing, surfing, swimming. The courses teach theory, history, and fundamentals of the subject. Some include practice sessions as well, in which the class canoes a fishing stream or dives for mussels. The classes are relatively inexpensive. Contact the adult education office of the school for more information.

Here you meet others with similar interests. You are no longer a romantic dreamer. Hearing friends express the same yearning to learn and experience nature, your notion gains substance. You are an adventurer about to embark on an exciting journey.

Fly-fishing Schools

Fly-fishing is an outdoor sport that is increasing in popularity across the United States. To some, it is an alternative fishing method; to others, it is the only way to catch fish, and to a few, it borders on a religion. The fly-fisherperson uses a long, willowy rod and artificial flies to attract and catch fish. The line and reel are matched to the fly rod in weight and balance. Together they form a smooth-working unit.

At this point, the student enters. Learning to cast the fly onto the water to a waiting fish is the first step. Fly-casting is an art, refined and exacting. It closely resembles cracking a whip. The rod is the base of the whip and the curling, stretching line is the lash. Unlike other forms of casting, it requires training to master. Orvis and Fenwick are two leading fly-fishing equipment manufacturers. Each founded a fly-fishing school for the purpose of teaching fly-casting as well as the finer points of fooling fish with an imitation insect.

In 1966, Orvis established its first school at Manchester, Vermont. Four years later, a second sprang up in Allenberry, Pennsylvania. At either location, the beginner as well as the advanced fly-fisherperson can participate in three days of casting, lectures, and catching fish. Lectures revolve around a color slide show that illustrates the relation between the kind of insects inhabiting a stream and the type of artificial fly to use. Tackle (rod, reel, line, and flies) is supplied by the school. Beginning in May, the lessons continue through August. Tuition is $135, including room and board.

Fenwick Fly Fishing Schools now number seventeen and can be found in California, Oregon, Colorado, Wisconsin, Virginia, Pennsylvania, New York, and Vermont. The main one, however, is the Montana-Yellowstone School in Fenwick, Montana. From June through September, the schools last three or five days. The three-day session involves two days of classroom work and casting instruction and one day of supervised fishing. Lunches and dinners are included in the $185 fee but not lodging. Two fishing trips—one by boat, the other by wading—are added to the basic course for the five-day school. The cost is $315.

Garcia Corporation is another fishing tackle manufacturing company that conducts seminars on fly-fishing throughout the country. A permanent school has not yet been founded. Instead, representatives travel to interested clubs or groups and teach the members fly-fishing.

Joan Salvato Wulff is one of Garcia's delegates and has been for twelve years. She has fished North America, Ecuador, Iceland, Great Britain, and the Virgin Islands. In addition, she is a former National Amateur and Professional Casting Champion. At age ten she "forced" her way into fly- and plug-casting with her father and brother. She watched and imitated and finally they offered suggestions and pointers to help her improve. But, for a grown woman, it is more difficult to learn an outdoor sport—especially a demanding one like fly-fishing—from a husband, father, or friend. As Joan explains it, "The average male angler wants every minute of fishing he can get out of his fishing trips. He doesn't want to have to 'baby sit' a companion." Especially a wife or girl friend.

Involvement with the outdoors begins with you. It would be idyllic for the man in your life to teach you about nature. But chances are, if he has the knowledge and experience, he does not have the time. If he has plenty of time, his patience quickly wears thin. If he possesses saintly patience, his motivation has disappeared. In short, the woman needs to depend on herself. Read the newspapers and find out about classes in the community. If you can afford it, attend a two- or three-day boarding school on fly-fishing or another outdoor sport which appeals to you. Some schools

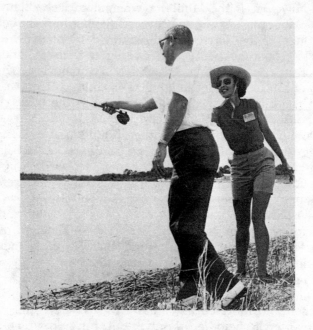

Joan Salvato Wulff conducts seminars on fly-fishing.

have women instructors but prepare yourself for being in a nearly all-male class. Women are shy about doing what they want, instead of what is expected of them. They confuse selfishness with broadening themselves. The first step in cultivating woodswomanship is learning something about the outdoors either in theory or by doing. Do it.

As more women display interest in outdoor sports, "ladies only" classes are being organized. Whether you agree with this concept or not, these courses educate women without the real or imaginary pressure of male criticism.

Bonnie Lilly is a twenty-six-year-old, native Montanan. She and her sister-in-law Annette Lilly conduct "ladies only" fly-fishing classes out of Bud Lilly's Trout Shop in

West Yellowstone, Montana. They emphasize casting, wading, knot tying, and knowing what trout like to eat.

Based on personal experience, Bonnie offers the following advice. "The first obstacle for a woman in the outdoors to overcome is not to lean back on the fact that she is a woman. She must learn to wade with authority—not mince along in pretty feminine steps. She must learn to cast for extended periods and ignore the initial muscle soreness. . . . We try to help women with the practical experience through our 'ladies only' program. We have found that women are much more receptive to learning fly-fishing from another woman. There is a mutual understanding of the problems encountered. Most women would like to learn to fly-fish so they

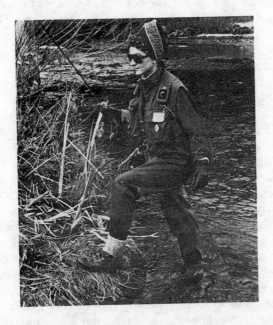

Fishing instructor Bonnie Lilly advises, "Wade with authority."

can enjoy the sport with their husbands, but the husbands haven't the patience to teach them. Our program is very flexible and geared to the particular woman we are teaching. Each session involves a maximum of two women, so it is very individual. In a nutshell, the attitude should be, 'If you want to do it, then do it!'" Annette adds, "While concentrating on the skill of fly-fishing, we try at the same time to share our enthusiasm about it."

Fly-fishing is more than catching fish. It is a strategy which involves knowing what the fish are feeding on and how to cast the artificial fly to make it look real. It is matching wits with the fish and trying to outsmart them. Anyone who says fish are stupid cold-blooded creatures has never outwitted one. You give them what they want in a way that looks appetizing to them. What if they are not hungry? Then, try to incite anger or rage. The "insult fly" is an effective bait because the fish strike out at it to remove it from their territory.

Besides the art of casting and the science of choosing the right fly to trick fish, fly-fishing is a philosophy about the outdoors. Catch-and-release fishing has become popular through the efforts of fishing groups, but especially fly-fisherpeople.

Catch-and-release suggests that fish are a limited but renewable resource. The fisher catches the fish and enjoys the thrills and heart pulsations associated with playing it. But then she returns the fish back to its waters. She releases it. This is vital for the future of fishing because there are increasing numbers of people who want to fight a natural creature with rod, line, and trained bodily reflexes. If each fisher kept every fish caught, the fish population would be drastically reduced.

The philosophy implies that nature is not to be used. It is not a precious mineral that can be purchased or spent. On the contrary, the untamed world has no price but is priceless. It offers no concrete rewards except the expansion of the spirit, exultation of the soul. Although nature can be felt, seen, smelled, and heard, its benefits are intangible.

With the privilege of actively participating in nature comes the responsibility of loving, protecting, and treating it with respect. Other groups of outdoorspeople feel the same way. But the fly-fishers have been the ones to organize this belief in a single concentrated effort called catch-and-release fishing.

Schools and seminars throughout the country teach every type of outdoor sport. Choose a subject you find genuinely interesting. Do not "force" yourself. If it sounds boring or ridiculous, no amount of instruction will change your opinion. If you feel guilty about leaving your family at night, enroll in a daytime class while children are at school and husband at work. Learn about the outdoors and seek a new horizon that broadens, not necessarily changes.

National Rifle Association Seminars

The National Rifle Association (NRA) sponsors seminars in many states. This agency educates and trains citizens in the safe and efficient handling of firearms. It helps concerned groups learn about hunting, backpacking, and other backwoods skills. Women In the NRA (WINRA) is a group of women dedicated to encouraging more active participation by women in outdoor activities. WINRA offers free lectures, film presentations, and brochures for women on hunting and conservation, wild game cookery, wilderness survival, and personal safety. For more information, write WINRA, 1600 Rhode Island Avenue, N.W., Washington, D.C. 20036.

WINRA's spokeswoman on backpacking is Sheila Link. She is an active outdoorswoman who writes about her experiences for newspapers and magazines and produced a weekly outdoor radio show in her home state of New Jersey. She believes that "any woman who really wants to, can learn outdoor skills. Short seminars are being offered in various locations all over the country and skeet and trap ranges offer instruction. . . . A gal can become knowledgeable about the outdoors on her own. My father wasn't an outdoorsman and, in fact, opposed shooting. He made me return to the seller a gun I'd bought 'on the sly.' My husband isn't an outdoorsman, either, but is instead a city boy and a scholar—afraid of horses, distrustful of guns, and totally disinterested in camping, fishing and canoeing. However, he does encourage me to 'do my own thing.' We've also encouraged our daughter and our three sons to do exactly what they want and each has chosen a different route."

It helps a woman to have companionship and emotional support from husband and children. However, if she does not, she can find a place for herself in the outdoors. It takes determination and practice but the woman who does becomes more womanly, more of a person.

OUTDOOR MAGAZINES AND BOOKS

A rich source of information and firsthand personal experiences can be found in outdoor magazines. Most of them are sold on newsstands or through subscriptions. Others are by subscription only. Begin with the ones in the neighborhood magazine display—those you have passed by until now. The magazines are segregated according to the subject matter. In some areas, they overlap. Stories about canoeing, skiing, backpacking, and camping knowhow can be read in almost any outdoor magazine. Read several and decide the ones you like best.

Outdoor Sports Magazines

womenSports is published by Billie Jean and Larry King. With the first issue appearing in 1974, *womenSports* aims to be the forum for sportswomen. In *Billie Jean* (Harper & Row, 1974), the well-known, outspoken tennis pro explains, "I don't feel the media give women athletes anywhere near the coverage they deserve, and that's one reason I've started my own sports magazine for women. . . ."

womenSports has promised to cover outdoor sports like jogging, hiking, backpacking, body surfing, and swimming. This magazine can provide valuable knowledge and a fresh way of looking at the outdoors and female participation. Information about workshops, seminars, and classes can be found there too.

Sports Illustrated is a well-written but slightly cynical

sports magazine. Its main emphasis is male competition on the professional and college level. However, more women-oriented articles are slowly being integrated into its scheme.

Outdoor Skills Magazines

Field & Stream, Sports Afield, and *Outdoor Life* are three national outdoor magazines available to the public on the newsstands. All have been written and advertised for men for over seventy-five years. Occasionally an article on game cookery is written by the wife of one of the male editors. But for the most part, women are left at home with the cooking, cleaning, and the kids.

A new trend has started, however. Margaret Nichols is now the Assistant Managing Editor of *Field & Stream.* Prior to the formal announcement in 1972, she acted as editor

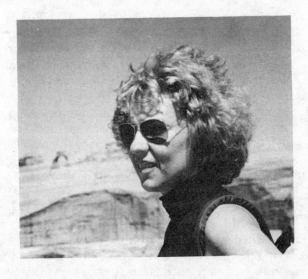

Margaret Nichols, Assistant Managing Editor of *Field & Stream,* writes a monthly column, "Especially for Women."

for the magazine but was listed under a male pseudonym. At last she can be credited for her work and monthly column, "Especially for Women." Few complaints have been received from the presumably all-male audience.

In *Field & Stream*, authors blend fact with an element of adventure for easy, fast, and often exciting reading. Photography is excellent.

Sports Afield changed its entire format in March, 1975. It is now a monthly outdoor encyclopedia. Everything you need to know about the subject of the month (in March, for instance, the featured subject is usually fishing), you can find within the magazine covers. Articles are short. Print is small. Illustrations outweigh photos. The magazine consists of the editors expounding on their specialty—for example, gun dogs, shooting, hunting, fishing. No women are yet on the staff. However, Joan Wulff writes an occasional article on fly casting.

Outdoor Life is packed with "me and Joe" adventure stories and colorful pictures of people, including women, basking in the outdoors. In October, 1973, Peggy Bauer was hired as the first woman editor. She and her husband Erwin became the wife-husband team of Recreational Vehicle Editors. (A recreational vehicle is a mechanical device used for recreation, such as boat, motorcycle, snowmobile, or travel trailer. However, in popular usage, Recreational Vehicle [RV] refers to a motorhome, camp trailer towed by a car, or a van in which one can temporarily live.)

Peggy writes from her home in Jackson Hole, Wyoming. She associated with the all-male staff of *Outdoor Life*—excluding her husband, of course—only at periodic meetings, usually held in New York City. How did it feel to be the only woman editor on the staff of an outdoor magazine? "The majority of men, I feel, treat me as an equal or a newcomer who they want to feel at home. All are gentlemanly; some even gallant. There is, however, also a strong feeling in some quarters that outdoor magazines should be *men's* magazines, written by and for men. I feel this is a business policy opinion, obviously not shared by the majority, and not a personal opinion of me."

But the policy won out. In July, 1975, *Outdoor Life*

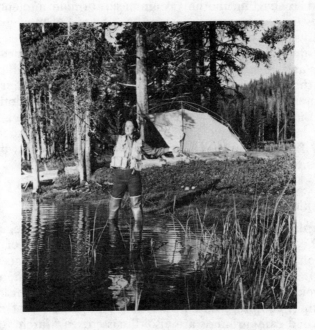

Peggy Bauer is an outdoorswoman living in Jackson Hole, Wyoming.—
Photo by Erwin A. Bauer.

dropped Peggy as an editor. The reason? "Who knows? I
sure don't." While Erwin moved from RV to Camping
Editor, Peggy was left out in the cold.

In this case, tradition won out over popular demand. On
the cover of the April, 1974 issue, Peggy was the first woman
ever to appear (but she shared the cover of *Outdoor Life*
with a man). Then, Peggy enthused: "This reflects the
growing interest of women readers." But now? "What's
probably the most encouraging sign to me about the present
trend is seeing young couples on the hiking trails with a
young baby riding right along. Not too long ago, the mother
would have been at home baking a cake, the baby in its

crib and Daddy pulling crab grass. How much better this way."

But *Outdoor Life* appears to have shut its eyes to this trend. By cutting the only woman editor from the staff, it seems to be attempting to stop the entrance of women and family to the outdoor scene.

Women should read the traditionally male outdoor magazines and voice their comments and preferences to the editors through letters. This is an effective means of pushing for more women staffers and preventing the indiscriminate exclusion of qualified women outdoor writers. These magazines are progressive enough to want to please readers, even if they are women. To effect change, the woodswoman needs to let her presence be known and felt.

Camping and Fishing Magazines

Camping Journal is the only genuine camping magazine on the market today. It features field test reports of new camping equipment. Articles revolve around places to explore and popular outdoor activities. At times, thought-provoking pieces appear concerning the philosophy of backpacking, camping, and wilderness. The problems of overcrowded campgrounds are also discussed. In March, 1975, Davis Publications (New York) expanded operations to *Backpacking Journal*. If your newsstand does not stock these two magazines, request them.

Fishing World, a by-subscription-only publication, deals with every aspect of fishing throughout the world. From Baja to Iceland, the articles read the same way a fisherperson speaks: full of tall tales, homemade theories, and secrets of the deep. Few female writers appear in print. More vocal female subscribers might change this. Keith Gardner, the editor, is progressive and highly imaginative. Write 51 Atlantic Avenue, Floral Park, New York 11001 for a subscription.

Wildlife Magazines

There is a long list of monthly magazines that feature the habits, current status, and future attempts to maintain habitat of wildlife. Almost every state fish and game department produces a monthly magazine for sportspeople and interested citizens. Pennsylvania, for instance, has two separate magazines—*Pennsylvania Angler* for fishers and *Pennsylvania Game News* for hunters. They inform the state population of new biological management techniques as well as describing the life cycle of a beaver or the appearance of a white-faced ibis.

Another example of a fine state wildlife magazine is *Wyoming Wildlife,* which publishes entertaining articles and excellent color photography.

National Wildlife and *International Wildlife* (534 North Broadway, Milwaukee, Wisconsin 53202) are two magazines, available by subscription only, that feature superb, closeup photography of animals. They deal with the beauty of the environment and how man sometimes thoughtlessly pollutes it, destroying wildlife in the process. There are a few instructional articles as well. These magazines keep the reader abreast of new developments in conservation and advise the citizen how to counteract undesirable, environmentally destructive legislation.

Audubon (950 Third Avenue, New York, New York 10022) is another outstanding conservation magazine. The photographs are of high quality. Intimate details of the life cycle of a whale or of a bighorn sheep can be found among the pages of this worthwhile publication. By saving each issue, a "living" encyclopedia can be developed. Here accurate information can be found concerning nature and wildlife and what man can do to improve both.

Books

The library is the first place to visit to learn about any subject, but especially about the outdoors. It has a varied selection of outdoor books written about all types of animals and birds, conservation, pollution, and outdoor sports. Even the books that have been published years ago are helpful. Conservation principles have changed little. Check out several books and study them. Familiarize yourself with important terms in your chosen field. Fishing, for instance, has a strange array of leaders, hook sizes, tippets, depth finders, pound test lines and rods, and types of retrieves. Learning the words is half the battle. Then you can understand what a fisherperson is talking about even though the actual performance is still a little puzzling.

Thousands of outdoor books are published each year. Usually, they do not receive as much publicity or as many key reviews as novels. However, interested readers can join a book club that features books on outdoor subjects. Publishers advertise these book clubs within the covers of the outdoor magazines. The *Outdoor Life* and *Field & Stream* book clubs promote books on hunting, fishing, outdoor cooking, and animal identification. This is a relatively inexpensive way to accumulate a top-notch outdoor library of your own. The novice can learn a wealth of practical facts from outdoor books. In most cases, the writing is good and the information is even better.

Outdoor book clubs advertise in outdoor magazines. Choose a book club that sounds attractive. You can practice tomorrow what you read tonight. Here are the addresses of the top two book clubs: 1) *Outdoor Life* Book Club, P.O. Box 2006, Latham, New York 12110; 2) *Field & Stream* Book Club, Harrisburg, Pennsylvania 17105.

CONSERVATION ORGANIZATIONS

An organization unites people with common interests and works for common benefits. The Audubon Society, the Sierra Club, the Wilderness Society, and the National Wildlife Federation are various organizations for conservation-minded individuals. Collectively, they wield political power. Repeatedly, they have demonstrated how united citizens can protect the environment by battling "big money" that finances strip mining and high-density development. Together people are strong. Individually, they do not have as much weight or influence.

Each of these organizations sponsors field trips and ecology clinics. Here representatives teach what their members hold so dear. By experiencing the outdoors, the novice understands why conservation is worthwhile and vital and why those who strive to destroy natural resources for profit must be stopped.

The address of each organization is as follows: 1) Audubon Naturalist Society, 8940 Jones Mill Road, Washington, D.C. 20015; 2) Sierra Club, 1050 Mills Tower, San Francisco, California 94104, with 45 chapters coast to coast; 3) The Wilderness Society, 1901 Pennsylvania Avenue, NW, Washington, D.C. 20006; 4) National Wildlife Federation, 1412 Sixteenth Street, NW, Washington, D.C. 20036.

Outdoor Women is a national organization for outdoorswomen. Here women unite to promote female participation in the outdoors. Workshops and seminars are offered to teach outdoor skills. Through Outdoor Women, manufacturers of waders, hunting gloves, boots, pants, jackets, and camouflage clothes are beginning to realize that there is a market for outdoor gear in women's sizes. Previously, these were available in men-only sizes. A woman would have to wear a small man's size.

Outdoor Women was founded by fifteen experienced woodswomen. They recognized a need for such an organization because many outdoor clubs do not welcome women. In fact, some bar female members.

Joan Cone is a certified Hunter Safety Instructor, a hunter and fisher. Author of *Easy Game Cooking,* she has lectured and demonstrated cooking, especially of game, throughout the United States and Canada. She was one of the first to formulate the idea of an organization for outdoorswomen. As she puts it, "Women are discriminated against outdoors. For one thing, we can not join Ducks Unlimited and certain Izaak Walton League Chapters. Many private gun clubs and sportsmen's groups are closed to us. Then, we can not compete in B.A.S.S. Tournaments and some other competitions. . . . These are reasons why we should get together as a national group and do something."

With headquarters in Washington, D.C., Outdoor Women is dedicated to action. Prior to its formation, a woman was dependent on men to learn, participate in, and fight for the outdoors. Now, she can consolidate her resources with other women to effect change, educate and create a place for outdoorswomen in sporting goods stores and fishing tackle and hunting gear shops. She can change her image from a lost soul out of her element to a capable, reliable, responsible nature participant.

NATURE OBSERVATORIES IN HOUSE AND YARD

Surround yourself with life: plants, fish, vegetables, trees, and birds. They divert your attention towards the growing segments of nature. They increase powers of observation. Little changes in a plant, for instance, are readily noticed on a day-to-day basis. Like humans, each living organism is somewhat different today compared to yesterday. To notice and record these alterations sharpen perception of detail—an outdoor skill that makes every moment afield even more enjoyable.

Houseplants

To a city woman, the closest connection to nature may be a plant. Perhaps you already have several. If not, purchase a few from a florist or grocery store. Identify each of them and learn about watering, feeding, and caring for them. They are more than ornaments. They are living, breathing chunks of nature.

To begin, rely on a book about plants for information concerning amount of sunlight, humidity, and warmth. *The World Book of House Plants* by Elvin McDonald (World Publishing Co., 1963) tells everything you want to know and more. It comes in paperback for easy reference.

After awhile, develop your own theories about the plants. You have lived according to secondhand knowledge long enough. Do it yourself and try to come up with your own answers. This is what self-confidence in nature is all about. In a small degree, you are living with nature when you adopt plants. They chip away at the cement curtain that is separating you from your origin in nature.

Terrariums

A terrarium is a specially designed arrangement of house-plants. It is simply a glass or plastic container filled with growing plants. Besides that, it can represent a beloved landscape or be planted to resemble a lush tropical garden. Using ingenuity and a smidgeon of skill, the terrarium can look like your favorite outdoor picnic spot or capture the mystery of cactus and desert. Terrariums need to be transparent to admit light, and waterproof to guard against moisture. Then, you can create a garden otherwise impossible under existing indoor growing conditions.

Brandy snifters, empty fish tanks, bottles, glass jars, and glass casseroles can be suitable sites for terrariums. Cover the opening with glass plates or clear plastic. Do not use a cover for desert plants, but most others thrive on humidity.

In making under-glass gardens, fill the container amply with rich soil. If the opening is too small to insert tiny plants, sprinkle in the seeds of the desired plants. As the seedlings sprout, use long, slender · tongs to remove the smaller, weaker ones. Within five to seven months, the garden will be in full bloom.

Bird Feeders

Birds are everywhere, even in the city. And they are always on the lookout for new places to feed. Put up a bird feeder. Within a short period of time, birds will be feasting right outside your window.

Bird feeders can be homemade or purchased commercially. The birds care less about how the feeder looks than about what it is stocked with. Commercially prepared bird seed is the best type of food until you become familiar with the birds and their likes and dislikes. You can then experiment with nutritious concoctions of your own.

Feeders usually attract perching birds. They are migratory; so from spring through fall, the feeder will likely lure many different types. These birds are wild. They are wary and cautious to ensure their survival. Erect the feeder on a pole about fifteen or twenty feet high. This way, the birds are out of reach of house cats, dogs, and other predatory animals. They are high enough to spot approaching danger from afar and fly away to safety. Place the feeder about fifty feet from the house. At this distance, the birds will be less jumpy about human intrusion.

For apartment living, hang the feeder on the patio or outside the kitchen window. If your feeder is birdless ten days after being set out, change its location. From a bird's view, it might be in a precarious spot.

Hummingbird feeders can be purchased at hardware stores. Fill them with a mixture of sugar, water, and red food coloring (dissolve one part sugar and two drops of coloring in three parts water). A long tube extends from the main bulb containing the food. The hummingbird sticks his long bill into the tube and extracts the nectar drop by drop. It hovers while eating with the wings beating so fast they are nearly invisible yet produce a humming sound. Hang the feeder outside of a window where you can observe the bird easily, for long periods of time. With fast aerial acrobatics and iridescent color, hummingbirds are fascinating. They can become fearless, swooping down and circling your head.

Hummingbirds are found throughout the United States. They are attracted by bright-colored, funnel- or tube-shaped flowers. Hummingbirds like honeysuckle, trumpet vine or creeper, morning glories, orange or red azaleas, tiger lilies and geraniums. They are constantly looking for a reliable food supply. Once the feeder is discovered by the birds, they will return each year.

Hummingbirds are special. They are the smallest of birds and can fly backwards, and yet when you watch them, you swear they have no wings at all. No matter how often people see them, hummingbirds are considered to be rare and extraordinary. Conversation stops when they appear at the feeder.

Bird Identification Books

"I wonder what kind of bird that is?" will inevitably enter your mind each time you see a bird at the feeder. The best way to find out is through a bird identification book. Many people who have never used such a book assume it to be difficult to read, requiring prior knowledge of birds. This is not true. *Birds of North America* (by Robbins, Bruun, Zim, and Singer; Golden Press, New York, 1966) is exceptionally helpful. With a little practice, you can discuss birds like an ornithological pro.

The knowledge gained from merely watching birds whets the appetite for more practical experience in the outdoors. You find yourself talking about plants and birds to your neighbors and friends. Surprisingly enough, they listen. You have tapped the basic world of nature.

Aquariums

The tranquility associated with watching fish cruise around in their own environment has long been a human pacifier. Whether the aquarium is simple and small with goldfish and guppies or large and complex with the limitless varieties of tropical fish, the effect is the same. You witness the life process of fish. Mating, laying eggs, hatching, problems of overcrowding. These living creatures are the world in microcosm. Their habitat is so unlike your own, you can not help but be engrossed by the fish activity. Human curiosity about fish is akin to the curiosity one feels about UFOs and outer space inhabitants. Go to the local pet shop and find out about aquariums. Choose the one for you.

Gardens

Build a natural world around you and discover how quickly it becomes part of you. A natural world, beyond indoor plants and birdwatching, requires a backyard or small plot of land. Size does not matter. Its fertility and what you do with the land is up to your natural inventiveness.

Build a wildlife garden by planting shrubs, bushes, and trees to attract small animals, like rabbits, squirrels and chipmunks, and birds. Provide natural homes for them. Cultivate a thick hedge of shrubs or a living fence of multiflora rose that is pleasing to look at and requires little, if any, upkeep. Buy a potted Christmas tree and plant it after the holidays. Pine trees not only beautify the landscape but shelter wildlife.

A more conventional plan for letting a bit of nature into your civilized life is by planting a vegetable garden. In no uncertain terms, working a garden brings you down to earth. A strong tie develops between you and nature. You till, cultivate, plant, and weed. But the magic is not in your hard work. It is watching the earth push shoots out into the open air. The vegetables from the garden enter your body, nourish it. You become part of the soil, the sun, the rain.

Long-range nature projects increase knowledge and appreciation of the wilds. They inspire a yearning to participate and live in the wilds instead of only observing. These projects help the rest of the family develop a sincere interest in the outdoors. Give each family member the chance to discover aspects of nature on his own.

Ponds

Water acts as a magnet for wildlife. The majority of animals and birds quench their thirst several times a day. They use the closest, most convenient, least dangerous waterhole they can find.

Set up a birdbath in the backyard and notice the number of birds and small animals that congregate there. The larger the body of water, the more wildlife it attracts. And if the pond sustains plant life and minnows, ducks, geese, herons, hawks, and ospreys might gather around it. A man-made pond can act much like a beaver pond in drawing communities of animals to it.

A pond of your own may be easier and less expensive than you imagine. It can provide recreation in the summer and can be stocked with fish. For a fishing pond, the minimum size is one-quarter acre. But for fun, it can be smaller. *Creative Fishing* by Charles Farmer (Stackpole Books, 1973) explains in detail how to go about it and how much it will cost. It is worth reading. A pond is an investment for the family as well as for nature.

At this point, you are gaining self-confidence. You wonder how you fit into the scheme of nature. You want to go out into the wilds and live there for a short time in harmony. Questions pop into your mind: Can I live in a less civilized environment? Can I do it? Me, the city girl? Yes. But there is only one way to convince yourself. Do it.

2

Minitrips

"On your own" is a challenge. Without help from husband, friend, child, you ready yourself to face nature. For gaining self-confidence, the only way to venture into the unknown is alone.

When was the last time you acted on your own? It is unusual to plan on being alone. Too often being on your own is confused with being lonesome. Actually they have nothing to do with each other. Loneliness signifies feeling abandoned, rejected, or neglected. It is a negative personal feeling. Being alone, on the other hand, is to be without companions. At a crowded party with people squeezing in from all sides, a person can feel lonely. Aloneness with nature, however, can induce a profound sense of peace.

Enter nature the first time by yourself and discover a heightened level of communication. Without distraction. Noiseless. Appreciation is simple and immediate. No explaining to a companion what you feel and why. Impressions register. Nerves relax. The mind opens and lets nature intermingle freely with brain cells.

While it is a good idea, it is not absolutely necessary to

be alone with nature. If apprehension descends at the thought of being alone in the wilds, take along an understanding and quiet friend.

Introduce yourself to nature through minitrips. A minitrip can be a short hike into a city, county or state park. It lasts one day or two, involving a one- or two-mile walk. It requires sound preparation but is less expensive than longer pack trips. The pack containing essential supplies is smaller and weighs less than the backpack used on maxitrips.

A minitrip can be a daylong journey, returning home by dark. Or it spans an entire weekend, camping out Friday and Saturday night. The initial contact with nature should be short, simple, and fun. Enough to encourage the hiker to return soon. By taking it slow and easy, enthusiasm will be throbbing and ready to go for the next time. On the first minitrip, venture off the main road early in the morning

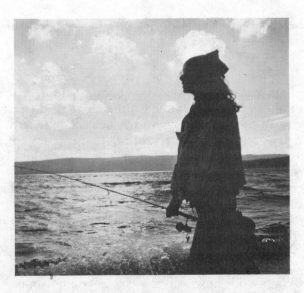

"On your own" is a worthwhile challenge.

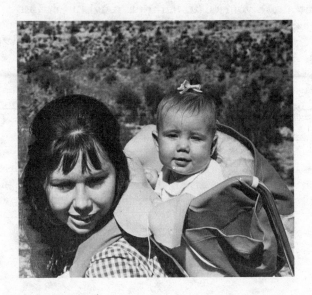

A minitrip can be meaningful with an appreciative, understanding friend too.—*Photo by Jim Tallon*

by foot or bicycle. Choose an attractive picnic spot. Later that afternoon, retrace the way back home at a leisurely pace. This is plenty for the first time alone in the outdoors.

A visit to the untamed world is not a haphazard affair. It can be exciting and surprising, maybe unpredictable. But to achieve a degree of relaxation without civilized luxuries, preparation is necessary. Preparing for the outdoors is the key to gaining self-confidence within this new realm.

"What do I want to do outdoors?" is the first question in preparing for a trip. The answer determines where you should go. Do you like long hikes or would you rather relax and soak up the scenery? Maybe wildlife photography or identifying wild flowers, plants, woodland mushrooms, or birds is your preoccupation. As an outdoorswoman, perhaps you prefer fishing, hunting, camping, and "roughing it" in general. Or you desire to escape from civilization without sacrificing the conveniences of home. Maybe you like to socialize with other campers and see the sights.

WHERE TO GO

The possibilities of where to go to learn or practice a favorite outdoor activity are endless. There are the mountains—the Appalachians, the Rockies, the Sierra Nevadas. If you like the water, how about the Great Lakes region, the Mississippi, the Missouri, the Columbia? Do not forget the innumerable ponds, streams, and lakes scattered across the country. The ocean and Gulf shores provide an unbeatable outdoor attraction. And the great Mojave Desert, teeming with specialized forms of life and mystery, offers an unusual yet interesting opportunity.

The amount of time and money available for an outdoor trip sets limits on how far you can go. For a minitrip, it is best to stay within familiar territory. But the choice is yours.

Wilderness and Primitive Areas

Wilderness and Primitive Areas are untouched by civilization. Motors are prohibited. Foot, horse, and hand-propelled boat power are the only sources of transportation. Hiking trails and spectacular scenery abound. Being relatively undeveloped, few camping facilities are available. Trails are usually well-marked and campgrounds may have outhouses. But piped water, picnic tables, and cooking grills are rare. So are a lot of regulations.

In September, 1964, the National Wilderness Preservation System was created by a presidential signature. This bill saved 9,925,352 acres of wilderness in 60 areas from development, such as commerical timber cutting, roads, hotels, stores, and resorts. Another 4,363,954 acres in 28 Primitive Areas are to be reviewed in the future as to their suitability for addition to the Wilderness System. These wild territories are managed by the Forest Service, a branch of the Department of Agriculture. Future additions to the

Wilderness System can be made only by Congress and then only after public hearings. In this way, wilderness is preserved as a national resource.

Most of the Wilderness Areas are concentrated in the western states—Washington, Oregon, California, Montana, Idaho, Wyoming, Colorado, Nevada, New Mexico, and Arizona. The Boundary Waters Canoe Area Wilderness in Minnesota, the Linville Gorge Wilderness and Shining Rock Wilderness in North Carolina, and the Great Gulf Wilderness in New Hampshire are exceptions. Primitive Areas can be found scattered throughout California, Idaho, Montana, Wyoming, Utah, Colorado, Arizona, and New Mexico. The Idaho Primitive Area, encompassing 1,224,733 acres of the Boise, Challis, Payette, and Salmon national forests, is the largest. Rugged, scenic, mountainous country with pure, fast-moving fishing waters and sleek big game animals are the main attractions.

Trying to explore a wilderness or primitive area on a mini-trip can be overwhelming. These wild regions are so vast that a weekend camper would only skim the surface. Countless opportunities greet the fisher, hunter, photographer, or hiker wanting to absorb nature. Seldom are other campers encountered. You are truly alone in a wilderness or primitive area.

Parks

In comparison with wilderness areas, the camping situation in the National Park System is tame, similar in many aspects to state and county parks. Organized campgrounds in parks usually offer modern clean restrooms, showers, picnic table, cooking grill, drinking water and garbage disposal. Some have full hookups for recreational vehicles—water, electricity, sewage. These provide a comfortable base camp for trailer travelers who enjoy other campers and desire conveniences. From here, sightseers can drive to historical, interesting park spectacles and nature programs.

Organized campgrounds are often sectioned off into "tenting only" and "hike in" camping spots. "Tenting only" means only tents can use that part of the campground. A

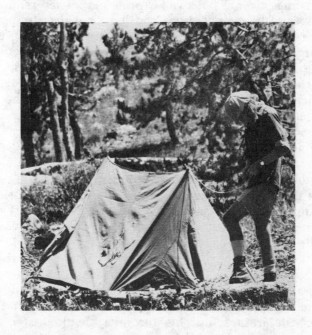

In "tenting only" sections of an organized campground, the camper can feel alone, deep in the wilderness.

hike-in campsite requires a short walk—500 yards to one-quarter mile. This is a controlled type of backpacking experience, valuable for novice backpackers who want to become acquainted with their equipment on a short, safe minitrip. But without backpack gear, the hike-in campsite can be demanding. It involves hauling supplies, tent, stove, cooler, and all other necessities some distance from the car. A nightly fee of approximately $3.00 is charged.

A park—national, state, or county—is ideal for a minitrip. The rules and regulations help the newcomer develop a sense of order—an initiation into campground etiquette. For instance, keeping a dog on a leash and depositing trash in the proper receptacle are two common-sense but un-spoken camping regulations. In addition, carefully tending a campfire and vacating a campsite without a trace of your presence are backwoods principles. They require the camper to be conscientious and harbor a deep respect for nature. With more and more vacationers setting up camps in organized campgrounds, each camper needs to cultivate a sensitivity. Litter or man-made scars on trees, grass, ground, and nature in general produces a shudder in the dedicated outdoorsperson. The more campers, the more vulnerable nature is to being trampled. The more careful campers are, the longer nature will exist in organized camp-grounds for others to experience.

Within a park camping area, other campers are close at hand, usually willing to assist in any difficulty. You can de-cide the level of "roughness" you want. Choose primitive tenting or civilized trailering. Cook over an open fire or use a camp stove. Pretend to be in the middle of nowhere or invite your neighbors over for a drink.

Miles of National Park backcountry are available for rugged backpack or horsepack expeditions. But these require at least five to ten days on the trail in order to do them justice. The experienced backwoodsperson can find such trips exhilarating. But the beginner should first discover the outdoors on a simpler, more elementary scale.

Commercial Campgrounds

Scattered across the United States are commercial camp-ing areas. KOA and Holiday Travel Park are two chains of commercial campgrounds. They offer game rooms, mod-ern restroom facilities, and full hookups for recreational vehicles. The charge is around $5.00 nightly. These camps provide a social structure for campers that many novices and some old-timers welcome. People are usually friendly and helpful.

Commercial campsites are like do-it-yourself motels. Places to park a camp trailer or set up the tent. From here you drive to worthwhile sights, fishing streams, or meadows of wild flowers. This type of camping relieves the strain on a thin vacation budget. A nightly parking space is cheaper than a motel room. The vacationer makes the initial investment in a recreational vehicle or tent and camping gear. After that, the trailer or tent becomes a traveling home. With such low overhead, a family can plan an economical vacation without sacrificing many varied outdoor experiences. The only drawback is that commercial campgrounds rarely assist in putting you in close touch with the wilds.

Private Land

Are you an independent person, who shuns order, signs, and directions? Would you rather go off by yourself than socialize? Then, all you need to become familiar with nature is a chunk of relatively unchanged land. Growing free and wild, this type of real estate falls under three categories: private, game and fish department, or Bureau of Land Management (BLM) land.

Potentially good private land for camping can be found in any rural section of a county. Always seek permission of the landowner or manager. Then, uncover the untamed, interdependent world of birds and animals. Photographic possibilities are everywhere. Wildlife flourishes in high brush and neglected field. Pheasants, grouse, quail, weasels, foxes, badgers, and sometimes deer are attracted to briar patches, overgrown hedges, and berry patches.

During late summer and early fall, treat yourself to strawberries, blueberries, chokecherries, huckleberries, and serviceberries. Plump, juicy, wild berries can be harvested in many parts of the country. The science of berry-picking starts with recognizing berry bushes. Before tasting, identify them. Even though poisonous berries are uncommon, they do exist. A local or regional flowering shrub or berry bush identification book is available at sporting goods stores or book shops. Paperback and compact, it is easy to carry into the field. Common berry bushes are pictured and described in two phases: the flowering stage and the fruit-bearing one, which lasts throughout the winter. For this reason, berries are important food for wintering wildlife.

During early summer, the beautiful flowering berry

bushes capture the eye. Mark the location of the bushes on a county or state map. Return later when the berries are ripe and heavy. Pick as many as you want. Pies, jams, and jellies can be made according to recipes found in natural foods cookbooks. Or the berries can be dried or frozen and used later to glorify pancakes or ice cream during the bleak winter months.

Berry bushes thrive in moist soil. Seasoned berry pickers claim that heavy snowfall in February and March and a rainy spring will produce a bumper berry year. On the other hand, a snowless winter followed by a dry spring forewarns a meager berry crop. During a good berry season, they say, a person can pick enough berries to last through a scarce one.

Game and Fish Land

Game and Fish land is owned by the public—you. It is managed by the state conservation department. This government agency is concerned with proper management of the state's wildlife. Agency personnel determine fishing and hunting regulations and stock fish and game birds in certain areas. Their goal is to provide good hunting and fishing to increasing numbers of sportspeople without depleting wildlife stock.

Most Game and Fish land is open to the public for hunting and fishing. Campers are welcome too. Some areas are close to home. They are patrolled regularly by game and fish wardens. This is where the beginner can find relatively good fishing. By combining this sport with camping, a closeness to nature can be experienced. It can change your whole frame of reference towards birds and fish. They, like you, are part of the natural cycle.

Game and Fish land sometimes offers the conveniences of restrooms, a wooden dining table, and stone fireplaces with cooking grill. However, the degree of campground development depends on individual state Game and Fish departments.

Check with the local office of the Game and Fish Department before the minitrip. Fishing seasons are set each year.

In addition, regulations controlling fishing methods and the number of fish that the sportsperson is allowed to keep are listed. If fishing is new to you, ask questions. The game and fish wardens are trained to answer and advise. Their job is to serve the wildlife resource and the public. They can tell you where as well as how good the fishing and camping are. They can suggest alternative areas where fishing is exceptionally hot or where a pair of ospreys have just built a nest.

BLM Land

The Bureau of Land Management (BLM) is a federal agency under the Department of the Interior. It administers public lands, located primarily in the western states, amounting to about 60 percent of all federally owned land. The overriding theme of BLM is multiple use. This includes camping and outdoor recreation, livestock grazing, mineral production, and maintaining fish and wildlife populations.

Even though such lands look uninhabited, they are full of life. Sage grouse, cottontail rabbits and jackrabbits, coyotes, feral horses, eagles, hawks, and many other forms of wildlife thrive there. By camping near a prairie waterhole, the photographer can be treated to a rich array of birds and animals.

BLM land is often vegetated with sagebrush. Sage prairies can be fascinating if the camper takes the time to hike and explore. Eagles perch and nest on the top of rocky buttes. Antelope graze on tender green shoots growing between the sagebrush. From flat-holed dens, badgers peer out with fiery eyes on alert for predators daring enough to tangle with these ferocious burrowers.

Camping on BLM or private land is primitive. That is, as primitive as you want it. You can park a self-contained travel trailer on a level spot of ground or you can set up a tent for a comfortable camp. Outhouses are usually absent. Running water, picnic tables, and cooking grills have not yet found their way into these forgotten parcels of nature.

Public or private, unrestrained, untethered land is ideal

for minitrips to test powers of observation. Wildlife finds
peace there and so may you.

Wildlife Refuges

For an extraordinary minitrip, one that focuses on wildlife
behavior and photography, bird and animal sanctuaries
are excellent. These are federal or state land set aside for
wildlife. Although visitors are allowed to walk along designated trails, the preserve is managed primarily for the protection of wildlife. It provides habitat, like marshes, which
are vital to the survival of many species but which are being
eliminated by encroaching civilization.

Within a sanctuary, animals act less wary, more accept-
ing of human intrusion. They sense that harm cannot befall
them there. With a field guide to bird identification in hand,
the experience can be unforgettable.

A refuge is not a zoo. Birds and animals are free to come
and go. Biologists use the preserves as natural laboratories.
From their studies, information about the habits and needs
of previously elusive birds and animals can be documented.
But unlike a zoo, a preserve protects wildlife natural to
that part of the world. For example, the J. N. "Ding"
Darling National Wildlife Refuge, stretching over much
of Sanibel Island off the coast of Fort Myers, Florida, is one
of more than 300 refuges in the United States, administered
by the U.S. Fish and Wildlife Service under the Department
of the Interior. There alligators, snowy egrets, the rare
roseate spoonbill, the threatened wood ibis, herons, ducks,
the bald eagle, and 270 different kinds of birds and 45
species of reptiles and amphibians can be found. Raccoons,
opossums, marsh rabbits, and armadillos also live in and
around the "Ding" Darling National Wildlife Refuge.

Camping is not allowed within the boundaries of a preserve. On the fringes, however, parking lots are often available for overnight trailer campers and nearby campgrounds
can be easily located.

Minitrips revolving around wildlife sanctuaries can transport the outdoorsperson to a prehistoric time, before man
changed the order of wild things and places. Untainted by

progress, refuges are magnets to living organisms. Here man is an intruder but accepted by the residents. It is humbling to realize that animals too have societies. They engage in conflicts and are influenced by the behavior of other animals. You leave with a new understanding that man is not the only creative, expressive creature on earth.

PRETRIP RESEARCH

Preparation involves finding out as much as you can about the chosen minitrip site before actually arriving there. Telephone or write the local Forest Service, national or state park, or game and fish office. Ask the representative specifics. What is the best time of year to see a variety of blooming wild flowers and mushrooms? When is the fishing especially good? How about the average temperature and amount of rainfall? When do most of the crowds of campers generally show up?

For a minitrip, research does not need to be extensive. But learn something about the area beforehand. Then, "You should have been here last month, the fishing was fantastic" will not be the response to a week of fishless fishing. Instead, you will be there during the peak fishing period. To many, research is a grueling ordeal. It need not be. Would you go to see a movie without first checking the time at which it began? Rangers, wardens, and information specialists assist campers. They can suggest nature trails that travel brochures may not mention. They spend a lot of time afield and if anyone knows about the attractions of the area, they do.

Obtain a detailed map of the nature tract chosen for the minitrip. Even if the planned destination is the local county park, a map can pinpoint trails and places of interest. Plot your course. Would you rather follow the stream or trek directly through the dense forest? Do you want to tackle hilly terrain or is the valley more your speed?

Knowledge of the area derived from personal contacts as well as from a map introduces you to the finer points of the place before you set foot on it. This is an important boost to self-confidence. Worries about what you might find

there are dissipated by facts. The location of the campground, its nightly fee, and its facilities are securely rooted
in your mind. How far your day-long hike will be and
approximately how long it will take you, have been tucked
away in your mental notes. You know the hour you will
start and when you will return home. The hard work is
finished. Now comes the fun. Pack and explore what you
have already acquainted yourself with through correspondence and personal research.

PACKS AND PACKING: WHAT TO BRING

Packing is exacting. The longer the trip, the more precise
packing must be. Why not throw a bunch of things into
the car and forget it? Because you will not have the car to
stockpile supplies. You only have one small day pack for a
minitrip; a backpack for a maxitrip.

A day pack is also called a rucksack. It is a small canvas
or nylon pouch with shoulder straps to hold it securely on
the back. Unlike a backpack, it has no aluminum frame to
help retain its shape. It is soft. For this reason, it is comfortable and when packed correctly, it can be worn yet
barely noticed by the camper. No strain.

When purchasing a day pack, consider all the items that
must be stashed inside it. On the other hand, you do not
want it to be so bulky that it moves from side to side when
you walk. In short, you want it big enough to carry essentials yet small enough to be an accessory instead of a burden.
Try on packs in the sporting goods store before you buy one.
If it is tight or confining empty, it will be more so packed.

Pack manufacturers (for example, Kelty, Eddie Bauer,
Medalist Universal, Gerry, Coleman, Camp Trails) produce many different types of rucksacks. Popular models
are constructed of urethane-coated nylon. This heavy-duty
cloth is waterproof, tear-resistant, and long-wearing. Look
for a YKK nylon coil zipper sewn securely into the bag with
nylon thread. Padded shoulder straps add comfort.

A waistband helps the camper distribute the weight in
the pack from shoulders to hips. Some packers like a waistband for holding the pack close to the body when bending

over for a cool drink from a stream or going through dense underbrush.

Day packs come in a variety of shapes, sizes, colors, and prices. Well-known, brand-name pack manufacturers can be trusted although their products are often more expensive. Also, the more comfort features built into the pack and the better the fabrics, the higher the cost. For a thorough survey of the packs on the market consult *The Master Backpacker* by Russ Mohney (Stackpole, 1976).

Basics

There are basics that an outdoorsperson should bring on any trip into the woods. Wooden matches—the kind that can be struck anywhere—are stored in a doubled sandwich-size plastic bag, twist-tied shut. Matches are fundamental to those who spend time afield. They are needed for the campfire. Through them, dampened spirits are elevated and outdoor meals are cooked. The ability to start a fire can be learned quickly, but not without dry matches.

An emergency supply of food should be included on a minitrip. Candy bars, a small bag of beef jerky, and several space sticks are essentials. These should be brought in addition to a lunch. Packing a plastic container of water, a canteen (the Army surplus kind is fine), or a thermos of hot chocolate is a good idea too.

In addition, elementary personal items should be carried. A roll of facial tissue makes fire-starting simple and comes in handy to alleviate a runny nose. A folding pocketknife can perform all kinds of outdoor chores from slicing a hunk of cheese into bite-size pieces, to introducing you to the art of whittling, to cutting stakes for roasting hotdogs over an open fire. In the backwoods, the absence of a pocketknife can be sorely felt when a need arises.

A waterproof windbreaker and a wool shirt are other "just in case" articles. They insulate a camper from the elements, inducing comfort, warmth, and dryness. Even on days that dawn warm and clear, temperatures can drop drastically with an approaching storm. It is best to be prepared.

Certain "cosmetics" can increase physical well-being in the backwoods. If you sufffer from parched lips, for instance, Chapstick can be a pleasant relief. Or extremely dry skin may require an on-the-spot application of moisture cream. Insect repellent guards against invading insects. Perhaps a painful hangnail screams for a clipper to trim it down to size. Small, seemingly insignificant aches and pains become large ones on outdoor trips, miles from conveniences. Examine the trifling discomforts that plague you at home. Multiply this by an inability to find relief in the rigors of nature. Then, promise yourself you will always remember the Chapstick, skin cream, nail clipper, or aspirin to alleviate the nagging irritation.

Extras

Pack the food, thermos, and basics in the day pack. What "extras" should be brought along on the minitrip? Sunglasses. A camera. Small, paperback versions of bird and wild flower identification books that fit easily into a rear pocket of your slacks.

Binoculars. A metal drinking cup. Chewing gum. A comb and tube of lipstick. A pencil for marking what specimens were found and where they were located. A bandana. A small nylon tarp for a picnic tablecloth and emergency shelter. A fishing rod and reel and a box of lures and fishing flies.

Not all of these things should be packed away. Binoculars and camera, for example, should be hung by a strap around the neck. There they are handy when you need them. Otherwise, good pictures and getting a closeup view of a bird or animal are missed. Shirt and jean pockets are indispensable packing spaces. Sunglasses and pencil go in the shirt pocket for easy access. The drinking cup can hook on the belt loop of your jeans. Comb and lipstick find a spot in another pocket. Scarf is tied around the neck. The fishing rod is hand-carried. Fit the rest into the day pack.

Try on the full pack. Too heavy? Eliminate an article or two. Packing for a minitrip is a series of elimination. Assemble the camp gear. Separate the essentials from the extras. Pack the essentials and include as many of the extras as possible. You soon discover how few items are needed.

ARRIVAL

This is the day. The children are in school. Husband, at work. House can be left for one day. Drive to the minitrip area. Check that you have brought everything you wanted. Put on the pack. Get out the map. Look at the time. Begin.

With the planning taken care of and the trail outlined on the map, you have time to enjoy the hike. Look around. Watch. Your pace is slow. Listen. Search for the little organisms that are everywhere. Smell the freshness of being on your own. Feel the vitality. Squirrels screech and scamper. They wait for your answer. Gray jays signal your arrival. A flock of green-winged teal splash across the water far ahead and take off in unison.

How does the trail and surroundings compare with what you learned from the map? Are you surprised? How long have you been walking? How soon do you estimate you will arrive at the picnic spot?

Select the perfect site for lunch. Be choosy. You can afford it. In all your dreams of picnicking alone in the country, what type of place did you imagine? Continue on the trail until it hits you, "This is the spot." Find what you want, what you are looking for in nature. You can do it.

PICNIC

Be comfortable. Spread out the tarp on a level section of grassy ground. Arrange the food on it. Relax and enjoy a leisurely lunch.

Would this also make a good campsite? You would need water. Look for a water source, such as a stream, spring, or pond. On a minitrip, you probably are not deep enough into the wilds for the water to be safe to drink.

Inhale deeply. Memorize the setting. Store it away in your mind. Then, you can recall the present moment whenever you want. The mere memory of this special place— you alone with the outdoors—will calm you.

Examine the wild flowers that you identified. Imagine the wildlife that relies on this piece of nature for existence. Can you see any signs of animals? Tips of bushes chewed off? Grass munched away? A circle of weeds pressed flat is evidence that an animal slept there recently. Animal droppings? Antlers that were shed by deer?

Savor every bite of lunch. It tastes different from food eaten at home. You are hungrier than usual.

RETURN

Glance at your watch. You know how long it took to reach this place. Should you leave now to return home at the appointed time?

The forest looks different now, as the sun is setting. You feel good. Are you anxious to get home or sorry you are leaving the outdoors?

You find yourself planning the next minitrip already. Where would you like to go? Your mind is relaxed. Everyday worries are sneaking back into your thoughts but they can be erased by absorbing the surroundings.

You did it. Congratulations. This is only the beginning.

3

Guided Trips

Smooth, rust-colored cliffs dwarfed the floaters. Overhead, the sun was a mere shaft of warm, hopeful light. The awesome slabs of stone were like the palms of two hands, guiding them swiftly towards disaster. Things were happening fast. The black, eight-person rubber raft bucked high on an angry brown wave, then plunged headlong downwards. Eight paddlers and their guide riveted strained eyes on the water beneath them. Bent with stress and determination, the team moved as much water as they could with the paddles. They hung onto the raft with powerful kneelocks on the air pontoons. Acting brave might calm the turbulence and prevent the cliffs from crumbling.

Mary Sue Rowan fought the river hard. Never before had she run a river—in fact, she could not even swim—but she had no time to think of such things now. Her right leg was submerged in mad, swirling water. The fifty-degree water incited her to dig the paddle deeper and pull it back with everything she had.

One wave stopped in midair immediately in front of the boat, demanding a reverent glance from its victims in the

raft. It broke over the boat, carrying the guide with it from
the bow to the stern. Mary Sue's sunglasses hung by only
one earpiece while she clutched the center rope. Being
washed overboard was vivid in her imagination.

The roar of the river seemed to quiet an octave. Everyone looked up to see if truly the end was coming up or if each
had lost the sense of hearing. Like a mirage, a calm placid
pool waited for them ahead. With the promise of peace,
the oarspeople spent their last reserve of strength. They
rounded a thirty-foot-high ominous boulder, made a sharp
right turn, backpaddled a little. They made it.

A common sigh was followed by silent, satisfied smiles.
Drenched and fatigued, they glanced around to give a
moment of homage to the mighty stretch of the Green River
they mastered.

Mary Sue is a housewife, living in Salt Lake City with a
husband and three children. Her husband Bob is a high
school football coach. Daily calisthenics, practice after
school, and weekend games during the fall keep him busy.
He is away from home much of the time. Their three daughters are engrossed with extracurricular activities at school.
Mary Sue frequently finds herself alone in their suburban
house—and lonely.

She sought a part-time job. But with a high school
diploma and no previous experience, the employment available to her was tedious and demanding, offering little personal fulfillment. Following her teenage daughter's example, she enrolled as a hospital volunteer. Depressing.

Quite by accident, memories of long, happy hours fishing at Greenwood Lake as a nine-year-old child in upstate
New York filled her thoughts. She had not touched a fishing rod since her family moved to Utah twenty-five years
ago.

Nellie Harms, a friend and neighbor, stopped by for
coffee. She had read about a three-day, guided float trip
down the Green River in the Sunday paper's supplement
magazine and was anxious to go. Would Mary Sue be willing to accompany her? "Sure."

Two rubber rafts departed Friday afternoon from Ouray
and arrived at Green River, Utah, Sunday evening. In be-

tween was Desolation Canyon, named by Major John W. Powell on July 12, 1869. He led a party of nine 1,000 miles down the Green and Colorado rivers in four wooden twenty-one-foot boats to the Grand Canyon.

Nellie and Mary Sue relived part of Powell's adventures. But it meant even more to Mary Sue. "For the first time, I faced water—my greatest fear. From now on, I can do whatever my mind is set to do. I am more confident in myself."

Self-confidence is admired. It makes a person worth knowing and befriending. It enlarges a woman's concept of the world. Life goes on outside the neighborhood and beyond her family. Self-confidence is the springboard to personal richness.

But to develop an unwavering belief in yourself, you need to know how to handle whatever arises. To achieve this, the outdoorsperson experiences the trying, challenging, exasperating, sometimes frightening. Without a guide or a teacher, it is doubtful whether these heights will be reached. Most humans do not like to push themselves to the limit. They want to maintain a safe margin between what they do and what they are capable of doing.

The value of guided trips lies in education. On them you can learn a special outdoors skill, like boat handling. Three different types of guided trips are available: 1) the weekend excursion, 2) the wilderness school, and 3) survival training sessions. Each of these places the individual in an unfamiliar situation. Alone, the person would not have ventured into this unknown realm. But with a knowledgeable teacher and plenty of companions, new circumstances can be faced and conquered.

THE WEEKEND EXCURSION

Guided float trips, horsepack fishing trips, and backpack photography trips that last three days or less are weekend excursions. The guides are usually self-employed, experienced outdoorspeople. They have a hard time tolerating the four walls of an office and have structured their lives to do what they like best while making a comfortable in-

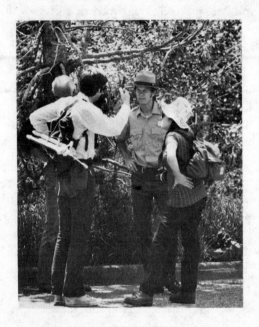

The value of guided trips lies in education. Here a park ranger guides a group on a photographic outing.

come. They often are superb storytellers and can be described enviably as "characters." They are natural leaders but prefer solitude. Cool-headed in crises, hot-blooded in arguments about dams, strip mining, and coyote control, they are usually practical conservationists. The newcomer can learn a textbook worth of knowledge by watching the guide.

Marlene Simons is a deer and turkey hunting guide in the Black Hills of northeast Wyoming. For twenty-three years, she has been stalking the woods to find game. Follow her in the crisp, frosty dawn November air. The cuffs of the slacks are tucked into the calf-high leather boots with rubber bottoms. On the balls of the feet, step gingerly among the colorful leaves and downfall timber. No twig cracks. Practically noiseless. Pause periodically and hold your breath. Listen for the thump of hoofs and the snap of a branch. Let your nose lead you to last night's deer bed. Slowly work your way to the top of the ridge. Search the dense growth with binoculars. Look for the glint of an eye, the flicker of an ear. No talking. Watch for telltale signs

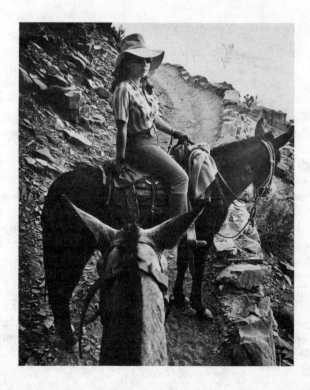

A mule trip into the Grand Canyon will never be forgotten.—*Photo by Jim Tallon*

of deer. Pellets? How warm are they? How far ahead are the deer? A nibbled juniper bud. A stripped berry bush. Subtle bits of information that tell Marlene where the deer are hiding and how soon she can expect to overtake them.

"I am a partner on the Windy Acres Ranch. I deliver calves, farm, put up hay and do a lot of our vet work. But I feel there is nothing more relaxing than a walk and a visit in the woods. The people who hunt with me, we work as a team. They take my orders and suggestions and listen because they feel I know my business. I honestly think they would not respect me if I did not do my job well."

To a guide, an outing is more than a job. It is personal pride. A never-ending test of backwoods skill.

Deciding on the Type of Trip

First, decide what type of outdoor travel appeals to you. River running or a scenic cruise? Fishing? The mountains or the desert? Backpacking or horsepacking? A relatively new kind of wilderness expedition is called the pack-hike. On a pack-hike, the camper walks five to ten miles each day but horses pack the gear. Each day guides do camp chores, set up camp at dusk in a new location, break camp in the morning and move on to the next campsite. In a sense, it is backpacking made easy. The camper gets plenty of exercise but without the strain of carrying a thirty-pound pack. Instead, a lightweight rucksack contains the day's necessities—lunch, insect repellent, tissues. While enjoying the benefits of walking through the forest, most of the work is eliminated. After a day's hike, you arrive in camp with the aroma of sheepherder's stew to greet you.

Guided trips are advertised in newspapers and magazines. The Sierra Club and national parks offer backwoods journeys. State game and fish departments or state recreation and travel commissions can provide a list of reputable guides.

How to Choose an Outfitter

The guided trip is increasing in popularity. As the demand rises, the consumer should exercise a degree of caution when choosing an outfitter. While most guides can be trusted, there are a few that cannot. Written correspondence is the best way to weed out the haphazard guiding business from the professional one.

Choose three or four appealing guided trips. Send a letter to the outfitters, asking specifics. For example, investigate cost, gear provided by them, items you should bring, probability of encountering bad weather, mosquitoes, black flies, or other pesky insects. What is the best insect repellent for that area? Is there a recommended level of outdoor experience and physical stamina? Are all meals provided? Can you keep the fish you catch?

The guide who answers your letter first and responds carefully can usually be considered the most conscientious. The tone of his letter, the cost and other information regarding the trip will tell you if this is the one you want.

Sleeping Bag

Some outfitters supply everything except personal clothing. Others, specify that campers bring sleeping bags. Either way, it is best to have your own sleeping bag.

The sleeping bag is probably the most important piece of camping gear. It insulates the body from the cold and lulls tiredness away into renewing sleep. Nothing is as refreshing as a dreamless eight hours of rest in the wilds. Nothing is as disturbing as a chilly, drafty, lumpy attempt at sleep. The difference between the two is a sleeping bag of high quality.

Sleeping bags come in a variety of shapes, sizes, and colors. They are constructed of different fabrics and stuffings. The general quality of the bag is reflected by its price. For instance, a good one costs around $60 to $100. This is a worthwhile investment for an enthusiastic outdoorsperson. Without a warm sleeping bag, the outdoors can represent a succession of restless nights.

Before purchasing a bag, consider where you will use it. On a backpack trip in the Arizona desert or a four-wheel drive journey into the Colorado high country. Desert nights in February can drop to a chilly fifty degrees Fahrenheit and summer evenings at high altitudes can be downright

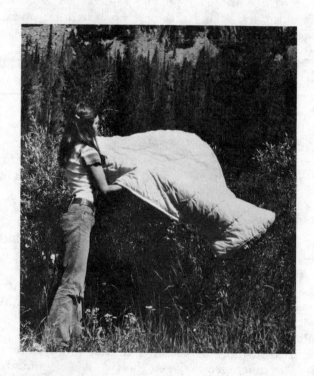

Bring a warm sleeping bag whether the trip is a weekend excursion or a
ten-day wilderness school.

cold—forty or thirty degrees Fahrenheit. Do not deceive
yourself by saying, "Oh, I'm just a summer camper. I won't
run into cold weather." Yellowstone Park can expose June
campers to a snowstorm.

A sleeping bag can limit your camping experiences. What
if old friends invite you to a rustic Wisconsin lodge for a
Christmas ski touring fest? Would you pass it up because
your bag could not counteract the 10- to 20-degree nights?

Comfort Range. The comfort range of a sleeping bag is the temperatures a camper can sleep in that bag without feeling cold. A comfort range of twenty-five to forty-five degrees, for example, is a fair all-around bag. But one with a range of ten to thirty degrees gives the camper more leeway. The lower the comfort range, the less chance of the outdoorsperson sleeping cold. When warm camping temperatures are encountered, the zipper can be left open, allowing ample ventilation. Being too warm in a bag is what many unprepared, shivering campers dream about but, in actuality, it seldom occurs.

Insulating Materials. The warmth or comfort range of a sleeping bag is determined by the insulation. The thickness of the stuffing and its ability to trap dead air, produce warmth. The insulation can be a type of polyester, found in most "summer bags." Another type is duck down. It tends to mat together, forming little balls of down which permit cold air to circulate into the bag. Drafts result.

Dacron Fiberfill II and prime goose down are two effective insulating materials. Prime goose down has been traditionally considered the best. Now, Dacron Fiberfill II has been developed and surpasses goose down in one important way. Prime goose down, when wet, balls up much like duck down. It is hard to dry and loses its insulative powers. Winter mountaineers discovered this drawback the hard way—on actual expeditions—and some suffered frostbite as a result. Paul Petzoldt, sixty-three-year-old mountaineer, worked with Dupont in developing Dacron Fiberfill II. It is designed to provide the insulation of down even when wet. Dampness does not mat Dacron Fiberfill II. And it is easy to dry. Paul Petzoldt Wilderness Equipment (Lander, Wyoming) manufactures Dacron Fiberfill II sleeping bags.

Goose down and Dacron Fiberfill II have good loft qualities. That is, the insulation is thick and springy. The fluffiness captures more dead air, which in turn produces more warmth. They can be tightly compacted into a stuff bag but, when removed from storage, will once again have their original thickness and springiness.

Goose down and Dacron Fiberfill II are both lightweight

insulators. The weight of the insulation is not as important as the amount of loft for warmth. Thus, both insulators are ideal for backpack sleeping bags. In weight, they vary from 4½ to 7 pounds.

Reputable Manufacturers. When comparing sleeping bags, it is wise to consider those produced by reputable manufacturers. They stand by their products and will fix the bag if faulty. Gerry (Denver, Colo.), Eddie Bauer (Seattle, Wash.), Paul Petzoldt Wilderness Equipment (Lander, Wyo.), and Alpine Designs (Boulder, Colo.) are leading sleeping bag manufacturers.

Shapes and Sizes. Bags are styled into two shapes— mummy and rectangular. The mummy follows the contours of the body, with no wasted space. It usually has a hood or drawstring around the top to help retain body heat. The rectangular, on the other hand, does not promote heat retention because of cold spots in the corners of the bag. But many campers prefer it. Instead of clinging to the body, the rectangular sleeping bag allows the sleeper freedom of movement. The camper can turn over inside the bag. Whereas the mummy bag turns with you.

Bags fit your physique—small, medium, large, and extra-large. The proper size is important. A bag that is too large means unnecessary air space which is harder to warm up. A too-small bag cramps the camper and interferes with sleep.

Zippers. YKK, full-length zippers should be sewn into a top-quality bag with nylon thread. A jammed or broken zipper can lead to nightmares. YKK zippers are heavy-duty with a nylon coil that does not freeze in below-zero weather. Full-length zippers insure better ventilation on a hot night.

Foam Pads. A sleeping bag is for warmth, but only does a fair job in smoothing out lumps and rocks on the ground underneath. For this reason, a foam pad is required. Major sleeping bag manufacturers design pads to go with their bags. A foam pad with a ripstop nylon covering can be three-quarters length, which supports the body from the shoulders to the hips. The bottom of the pad should be covered with a urethane-coated nylon that protects bag and sleeper from moisture.

To an outdoorsperson, a quality sleeping bag is like a pet dog you would not sell at any price. It is a best friend. It soothes away the day's aches and pains with soft, tender treatment. It does not talk back and has a lifespan of ten to fifteen years if treated well.

Other Necessities

Guides at times take a lot for granted. "We supply everything" may be the answer to "what items should I bring." It slips their mind that this may be your first venture into the backcountry. They assume you know what the essentials are. But most newcomers do not.

River Running

On any type of boat trip, but especially river running, canvas or nylon tennis shoes should be worn at all times. Your feet will inevitably get wet. Gym shoes dry fast and yet provide traction on a slippery deck or rocks.

River running implies that the rubber raft will encounter fast water and occasional high waves. Large waterproof duffel bags contain all gear and are lashed to the bottom of the raft. This insures nothing will be thrown out of the raft. For double protection, bring along several heavy-duty giant-size plastic bags. Wrap your sleeping bag, camera and extra clothes in one of the plastic bags. The guide will store it in a duffel bag. Too often, these duffel bags spring leaks, soaking all the gear not stored in waterproof plastic. Lying in a wet bag is like curling up in a puddle.

Bring a bathing suit, suntan lotion, and a wide-brimmed hat to protect the face from too much sun, and polyester blouses and shorts that dry quickly. Also include a pair of jeans, a wool shirt, and waterproof windbreaker which act as shields from the elements. Do not wear socks while on the river but pack several pair of wool socks. Nights on the riverbank can be cool.

Horsepacking

A rider who spends several hours in the saddle wears long slacks. Novice horsewomen with sensitive skin should wear long underwear beneath slacks. Denim jeans, traditionally the cowgirl garb, are rough on skin and can hasten the appearance of blisters on knees or legs. Slacks made of heavy cotton without bulky seams meet the needs of the beginner horsewoman. Sitting straight in the saddle, putting most of the body weight on the legs and stirrups, also minimizes saddle soreness.

A wide-brimmed hat, insect repellent, and raingear, carried in the saddlebags, are necessities. Boots should be worn to protect ankles from blisters. In addition, experienced wranglers advise that the boots should have a well-defined heel to prevent the foot from slipping completely through the stirrup. Although this is probably true for riders who are breaking a horse, herding cattle, or roping calves, it is not a must for the novice. Many horsepack trips occur during the rainy season. Wear boots with rubber bottoms to guard against moisture. Cowboy boots are fine to wear in sunny weather when most of the time is spent in the saddle. For the person who wants to get off into the woods, a comfortable pair of hunting or hiking boots is best.

On a horseback fishing trip, pack the rods in a sturdy aluminum case and tie it onto the saddle. Specialized backpack rods that break down into a case twelve to twenty-four inches long are best. Large aluminum rod cases seem to spook high-strung horses.

Put accessories you will need in the saddlebags. These include fishing reels and lures or flies, identification books, lunch, and a thermos of lemonade.

Hiking Trips

Tackling large expanses of backwoods on foot is exhilarating and fun. But not without correct footwear. Good hiking boots prove their worth in terms of ankle support, blister prevention, and general massage of the feet.

Hiking Boots.   Hiking boots are not mountain climbing boots. Mountain climbing boots are of heavyweight construction, weighing four to six pounds a pair. They are built with extra padding and sturdy materials, designed for rugged use. Inflexible, they are difficult to walk in for any length of time.

Hiking boots, on the other hand, are a lighter boot—lighter in construction and weight (two to four pounds per pair). They cost less too. Being less bulky, they facilitate long hikes. Hiking boots have Vibram or lug soles for better traction. Made of leather, they can be effectively waterproofed with Sno-Seal, Mink Oil, or a similar substance. They cover the ankles and have laces from the toe to the ankle; speed laces are convenient and save time. Hiking boots are padded and seem clumsy at first. However, they should not feel uncomfortable in the store. Wear two pairs of wool socks when trying them on. They should fit rather loosely, not snugly. Extensive walking swells the feet. Two pairs of wool socks protect feet from moisture and blisters.

Most top-notch hiking boots are made in Europe and cost $30 and up. But they can last a lifetime with periodic resoling and frequent reapplication of waterproofing.

"Breaking in" a pair of hiking boots is not as painful as it is with many dress shoes. It is a matter of wearing them an hour or two daily three weeks before the trip. Because of the reinforced construction, your foot conforms to the boot instead of the other way around. A hiking boot does not crease like other shoes and beginners occasionally feel that their feet are being constricted. In truth, they are being safely supported. The hiker merely digs the toe into snow, mud, or dirt and walks up a steep grade without slipping. To descend mountainous terrain, the heel of the boot is thrust into the snow or ground for sure-footed balance.

THE WILDERNESS SCHOOL

A wilderness school is a ten-day to two-month course taught by knowledgeable instructors, using the outdoors as a classroom. Basic curriculum deals with conservation practices, that is, teaching wilderness users how to enjoy an area yet leave it in its natural state. The education is practical. No textbooks. The student learns each day by doing. In addition, certain outdoor skills, such as backpacking, ski touring, fishing, and mountaineering, are taught. A person, ignorant of nature, can enter a wilderness school and emerge relatively skilled in outdoor activities. The basic philosophy is respect for the outdoors through appreciation for what you can do there and the benefits derived from it.

The National Outdoor Leadership School and the Outward Bound School are two leading wilderness schools.

The Outward Bound School

The Outward Bound School philosophy began in 1942 as a crash survival course in Wales for merchant seamen. A certain blend of experience and challenge prepared the men physically, mentally, and psychologically for the hardships of war. The men compiled a remarkable success record during World War II. They attributed their success to their training.

Over the years, the emphasis changed from survival to personal growth. The first American Outward Bound school started in Colorado in 1962. The goal was to teach young people values and develop an undefeatable spirit within them. The program exposed them to nature and the elements and taught them how to cope.

Now six independent Outward Bound schools are located in Colorado, Maine, Minnesota, North Carolina, Oregon, and Texas. There is also a Dartmouth Outward Bound Center at Hanover, New Hampshire. Each school utilizes the natural resources found in its respective part of the country. The Maine Outward Bound School, for instance, is situated on Hurricane Island, ten miles off the Maine coast. There seamanship, navigation, and ocean sailing expeditions are the main courses.

The basic twenty-three-day Outward Bound course taught by the Colorado school, the largest in the United States, involves backpacking and rock and mountain climb-

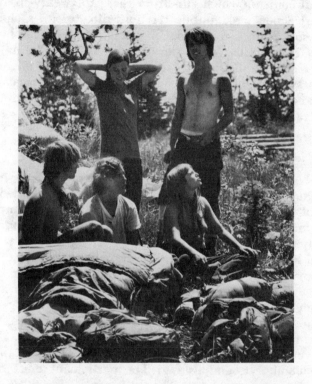

The wilderness school teaches practical outdoor skills in the open air classroom of nature.

ing. Care and protection of the environment, first aid, field
food planning and preparation are part of the program.
Towards the end of the course, each student undergoes the
Solo. That is, the person takes food, clothing, and shelter
into the wilderness alone. Without company, the student
stays within a certain area until the instructor comes. It lasts
about three days.

As one student described it, "The physical challenges of

Outward Bound taught you things you needed to know about yourself, stripped away masks and fears, gave you a new sense of confidence."

In addition to the standard course, Outward Bound offers special courses, which run from three to twenty-six days. Robert Schenkeink, public relations director for Colorado Outward Bound, reported, "A special program for housewives is currently being developed. We hope to have it open to the public soon." Programs are presently offered to business executives and school teachers. A four-day raft trip and a ten-day desert Utah trip are the most popular. Cost ranges from $200 to $450.

The National Outdoor Leadership School

The National Outdoor Leadership School (NOLS) headquarters in Lander, Wyoming. Paul Petzoldt founded the school in 1965 to combine conservation, winter camping, and mountaineering into a united, coordinated course of practical study. Instructors stress leadership. Students take turns leading a small group. Eventually, they travel in a group without an instructor. The appointed leader is responsible for setting the pace, route finding, and maintaining safety.

The wilderness expedition is the basic NOLS course. During thirty-two days in the mountains, the enrollee gleans an overall knowledge of the fundamentals of mountaineering, woodcraft, and fishing. The participant must be at least sixteen years of age. The tuition in 1975 is $650.

Relatively new, biology expeditions are summer schools in the field. They offer university credit in biology and natural resources. Students learn about ecosystems while actually taking part in the whole scheme. Most of the expeditions take place in the Wind River and Absaroka mountain ranges of Wyoming. However, there are branch schools in the Pacific Northwest, Alaska, Utah, Baja California, and Africa.

A highly publicized NOLS event is the annual Christmas ascent of Grand Teton Mountain in northwest Wyoming. The expedition attempts to reach the top of the Grand by

January 1, despite 60 to 100 mph winds, frigid temperatures, and deep snow.

Other mountaineering schools exist throughout the country. They teach the interested person how to live in the rugged wilds while mountain climbing. The two go hand-in-hand. To become proficient at the demanding, strenuous sport of mountain climbing, a person must also cultivate a profound veneration for nature. Stressful outdoor classes are designed to reveal a broader, full-of-potential new you. They demonstrate how interdependent humans are on each other and nature.

The wilderness school is not for everyone. To some it is an irresistible challenge. To others, the height of physical and mental achievement is to stand on top of a mountain. But do not be mistaken. A person need not be an excellent athlete in superb physical condition to be a mountain climber. Average physical conditioning is all that is necessary.

The major factor is the mental frame of reference. You want to climb that mountain no matter how afraid you are. You are willing to accept hardships to get there. Pessimism, cynicism, or giving up is out of place. Knowing that thousands have already accomplished what you are trying to do can help. By the time you reach the summit, a firm belief in yourself will envelop you. With a goal in mind, you reached it. The wilderness school can be means of acquiring deep faith and confidence in oneself.

SURVIVAL TRAINING SESSIONS

Enter the field with only the clothes on your back. Live without the aid of any manufactured item. Obtain your food from the land. Build a shelter for yourself. Construct a variety of hunting implements and bag game with them. In short, enter with nothing, use what is available, and leave with your life and a good story.

The survival training session is designed to prepare a person to cope with emergency situations where nothing is available except what can be found in nature. This is an extreme circumstance that can be dangerous. Especially if the student is not mentally or emotionally mature enough to handle it. Survival training appeals to some people, a minority. With others, it bolsters a sagging ego.

The Highland Survival School with the head office in Colorado Springs, Colorado is one of the best. Larry Dean Olsen, author of *Outdoor Survival Skills*, is one of the directors. In 1967, he established a program at Brigham Young University entitled "Youth Rehabilitation through Outdoor Survival."

Richard Jamison, another director of the Highland Survival School, himself says that after evaluating "several survival schools in the country, it is my opinion that many of them are doing an injustice to the students they teach. . . . Many of the so-called survival schools should be renamed 'camping schools.' They dangerously lull their students into a false sense of security. He tells himself, 'I can survive. I have attended x number of classes at a bona-fide survival school. I have a survival kit.' Then, when an emergency situation actually arises, the student has had no actual experience and finds himself ill prepared to cope with the problems which will arise both physically and mentally. . . .

"On the other hand, survival schools that teach their students to be self-sufficient are extremely beneficial both to the experienced outdoorsman as well as the novice. It has been proven with over 2,000 students at Brigham Young University that learning to be completely self-sufficient can help the student attain many personal goals as well as raise the academic grade level."

A major goal of survival training sessions is to build self-confidence. But survival training, dealing with life-or-death situations, is an extreme in itself. Self-confidence can be gained through weekend excursions or more demanding wilderness schools where enjoyment is stressed first, overcoming physical obstacles, second.

Prevention is the best defense against facing a survival situation. The outdoorswoman who knows how to prepare for a trip can foresee and prepare for emergencies before they happen. Even in natural disasters, such as a flood or plane crash, rescue teams are dispatched immediately. The

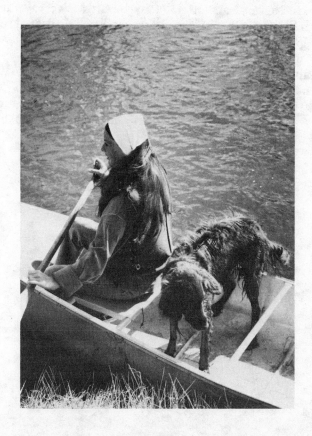

A new sense of self-confidence develops with wilderness expertise.

self-confidence gained from enjoyable contacts with nature will carry over to an emergency situation. Sound judgment and knowledge of basics—like how to read a compass or follow natural landmarks, how to build a fire, how to stay warm—will ward off panic.

The survival school has its place. But teaching self-confidence is not its fundamental goal. Rather, it is to teach its students to survive with nothing. In addition, survival may be so rough on the body and spirit that the student may disavow the outdoors later. Nature is to enjoy. To exist there as an animal may be attractive to some but not to the majority. Be careful in choosing a survival school. Its reputation should be investigated thoroughly. You have a lot at stake.

Gaining self-confidence is the key to another world and a broadened you. It opens the door but it is up to you to walk in and extract the spiritual riches waiting for you there. You must take the chances and explore the unknown. The rewards will follow naturally.

4

Retaining Femininity

According to Western folklore, the rugged outdoors transforms a boy into a man. But what does it do to a girl? Can exposure to the rigors of nature make a female manly? Today's society says, yes. Little girls who climb trees, collect frogs, and fire BB guns, are labeled tomboys. Well-meaning aunts, cousins, and older sisters hope for the day when their beloved tomboy "discovers boys." Then, she will lose interest in the outdoors and become preoccupied with hairdos, clothes, and makeup. Or will she?

Adults unconsciously divide the world into two parts. The outdoors—cutting the lawn, painting the boat, and washing the car—belongs to males. The indoors—house-cleaning, making beds, babysitting—is the female realm. Even though the male and female territories overlap, the responsibility for outdoor upkeep and care lies with the boys and men of the family. Furthermore, once the chores are done, the men fish, pitch horseshoes, or golf.

Women and girls, on the other hand, are expected to be knowledgeable about indoor appliances, cleansing agents, and keeping drains unclogged. After their jobs are completed, they sew, read, or play bridge.

THE TOMBOY CONCEPT

The division of labor between men and women, boys and girls, is largely determined by society. The way men act reinforces the fact that they are of the male gender. Similarly, women are expected to act in a female manner, which is limited mainly to home, babies, and volunteer work. Based on this type of thinking, a career woman who works in the outdoor field should have been a tomboy as a child and should be a bit on the masculine side—"a tough old boot," as some westerners put it.

To test this theory, twenty women, who have achieved notable measures of success in the outdoor or athletic field, were interviewed. Each was asked how she first became interested in the outdoors and if she were ever a tomboy. Out of the twenty, eight said they were never tomboys, seven admitted that they were, and five refused to answer the question.

Marty Stribling, a twenty-eight-year-old public information specialist for Cibola National Forest, Albuquerque, New Mexico, explains the dilemma that many girls and women face. "My mother was picking apples the day I was born. As a result, I almost had my first breath in the out-of-doors. I grew up with parents, grandparents, five brothers and a sister who are all earth-loving individuals. We shared many memorable hours near mountains, bright water and open skies.

"We left the farm for the city when I was six as it was difficult to make a living as a farmer, even then. Economically things were better. But all of those everyday natural things I had done in the country were suddenly given new perspective by city neighbors. They said little girls are different from little boys and should wear a dress (to climb a tree?) and have clean knees, curls, bright manners and sterile minds.

"For the first time in my life I was given a name unfamiliar to me. I was called a tomboy. Fortunately for me, I was a strong-minded individual and so was my mother. I continued to climb trees, ride bikes, build sandcastles, run, jump and grow naturally, enjoyably and sanely. As a result, I have a lot of good judgment and my own reality. And to some, I am still a tomboy."

The concept of tomboy is mainly suburban. There children participate in organized activities: one set for boys and another for girls. In less structured communities where fun is up to the kids, girls and boys play together without discrimination. Without learning otherwise, children devise games they all like and can play, regardless of sex.

Apparently being a tomboy as a child has nothing to do with a woman's choosing the outdoors as a way of life. The group of outdoor women interviewed was evenly divided between those who had been tomboys as children and those who had not. However, they expressed similar attitudes towards the outdoors. None of them considered the outdoors exclusively a man's domain. Nature attracted them and they followed. Each of them thinks of herself as a person rather than as a woman. The possibility that certain areas might be out of bounds for women never occurred to them.

MODERN OUTDOOR WOMEN

Modern outdoor women can be characterized by an independence of thought and action—"my own reality," as Marty puts it. They are doers and welcome the chance to test their know-how. They shun passivity and timidity. They seek the unknown and the challenge.

Jane Baldwin is a good example. She was the first female backcountry ranger in Grand Teton National Park, Wyoming. Born and reared in Bakersfield, California, she was casually interested in the outdoors but did not have an opportunity to delve into nature until 1969. At that time, she learned backpacking and rock climbing from friends. "I realized that more men than women were interested in the outdoors, but that happened because they had always been encouraged in that direction. Women had been encouraged in arts, crafts and home economics. More women should be helped to pursue outdoor interests. Then, they could experience what I have. It would be great for them."

During the summer of 1974, Jane was the first woman ever to assist with the actual rescue of an injured mountain climber in the Grand Teton mountain range. A young male climber broke both ankles in a fall when a boulder he was

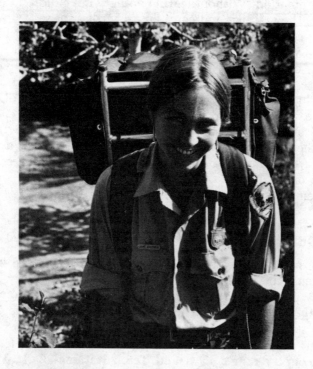

Jane Baldwin was the first female backcountry ranger in Grand Teton
National Park, Wyoming.

scaling suddenly broke off and rolled down the mountain-
side with him on it. A total of eighteen rescue mountaineer
rangers worked three days to transport the victim down the
mountain and to the hospital in nearby Jackson, Wyoming.
    The eighteen rangers were divided into three litter-carry-
ing teams. One team of six persons would haul the litter as
far as they could. Then, the second team would take over.
While the second team rested, the third would assume responsibility for the litter. The three teams rotated in this

fashion for three days until the victim was safely off the mountain.

Jane, who is 5 feet 8 inches tall, weighs 122 pounds and is 24 years old, carried her weight in the rescue continually for 20 hours. Quiet, with long brown hair, opal eyes that look through you, and a quivering smile, she looks like she could be a librarian. She appears gentle, sensitive, and especially vulnerable to criticism. Yet she successfully participated in an endurance struggle with an all-male team of rangers to rescue an injured climber.

As a backcountry ranger, she backpacks a distance of about five miles to Surprise Lake, sets up her tent, and lives there alone five days out of every week. During the second week in July, the thick layer of ice that seals off the lake most of the year finally thaws. As a primitive substitute for a bath, she swims briskly in the frigid water for a few minutes once or twice a week. "It's invigorating but the water is so cold you can hardly breathe. When swimming at an elevation of 9,540 feet, it takes longer to get the circulation going again than it does to dry."

Within Grand Teton National Park, backcountry visitors camping in areas above 7,000 feet are not permitted to build campfires because of the scarcity of wood above timberline. Jane cooks over a white gas, single-burner stove. She packs all garbage (including used toilet paper) in a large, heavy-duty plastic bag and carries it back to civilization with her. Three backcountry rangers are assigned to a section of wilderness where a patrol cabin is available. Here the ranger lives for five to ten days. But Jane is one of three delegated to manage an area that does not have a permanent place of residence. Instead, she lives in her own two-place backpack tent.

There is an epilogue to the mountain rescue feat. Jane arrived home at 4:30 A.M. and fell into bed exhausted. The next day, she brought freshly-made chocolate chip cookies to the injured mountaineer, recuperating in the hospital with both legs in a cast. Another ranger who also was on the rescue team accompanied her. The victim cheerfully remembered Jane, despite his groggy condition, and welcomed her. However, he did not recognize the male ranger.

"Over the 20 hours I helped carry the victim down, I had to remind myself several times that inside the litter was a suffering, uncomplaining human being who must feel worse than I did, even though I was completely fatigued. I was so tired I felt myself fighting for survival. But I directed my thoughts to the rescue and that a man relied on me to get him down to a hospital." Somehow, she communicated these feelings to the injured climber and he was grateful.

DEFINITIONS OF FEMININITY

Femininity is how a woman sees herself. It is not lace, ruffles, and petticoats. It is brushing your hair, washing your face, standing straight, walking in graceful strides, sitting at ease. Wearing curlers and face cream to the supermarket is announcing to the world that you are tired of being female and want to be neuter instead.

Femininity is the ability to rise above present problems and to project an inner calmness over those around you. It is a process always going on, refining itself, becoming more natural. Feminine minds tend to see the subtle, read purpose into happenings, and search out beauty and meaning. As Joan Cone (see Chapter 1) puts it, "I think that femininity consists of a certain outlook on life which we girls have. It isn't something one can explain. Going out and sitting in a duck blind in the rain. Then, coming in and putting on blushing pink lipstick. How can you explain it?"

Nagging, complaining, and feeling queasy, squeamish, or faint are tricks to get your own way. Many women ride along in a fishing boat with their husbands but do not fish. Or they wait in the car while their husbands hunt rabbits. These are the ones who sometimes use negative verbal comments to express boredom or a lack of understanding about the outdoors. They nag or complain out of habit more than out of malice. Yet the effect is the same. They irritate their husbands or friends to the extent that they will not be welcome to accompany them on future fishing or hunting trips. They will be left home alone. These are the women who should venture out on their own and test their own abilities to meet the challenges of nature.

Involvement is the only cure for nagging and complaining. Attention is diverted away from yourself. You concentrate on casting a lure to a certain hole, finding rabbit tracks in the mud, or scouring the countryside for a fossil. Spectator sports may prime the disinterested party to criticize. Being an armchair quarterback is for the very old, the physically disabled, or the skeptic. Active participation, on the other hand, keeps one young and alive.

To Bonnie Lilly (see Chapter 1), "femininity means 'soft.'" Not weak or wishy-washy. Not impotent or ineffectual. To Bonnie, soft defines an emotional approach to people, especially to those she loves. In this regard, soft means malleable to the desires of husband, friend, or family. If the idea of venturing into the outdoors is frightening or discomforting, sacrifice yourself for the sake of the one who wants to share with you. A ready teacher is exceptional and invaluable. Accept the offer lovingly and do not question your ability to learn and become part of nature.

Remember, society has traditionally barred a woman's involvement in the outdoors. Since childhood, you have been trained to think you are too weak or too pampered to face and actually enjoy the trials of nature. Years of conditioning have tried to convince you that your place is in the home. Accept nature's invitation and see for yourself.

As Jane Baldwin advises, "Never doubt your abilities in the outdoors. You'll almost always surprise yourself at how well you do, especially if you approach things with some self-confidence. Don't spend time with men who aren't willing to give you the same chances they had in becoming familiar with the outdoors." Jane knows what she is talking about. She learned mountain climbing from friends; she never attended a class. And each time she approaches a mountain, a fear of heights fills her stomach with dread. She overcomes this disabling fear through confidence. She believes she can do whatever she puts her mind to. This she has proven. So can you.

HOW TO FEEL FEMININE OUTDOORS

Outdoor clothing manufacturers are not yet aware that a great number of women are avid fishers, hunters, outdoor photographers, and campers. As a result, fishing waders and vests, camouflage jackets, hunting gloves and vests and other types of sensible outdoor clothing such as wool shirts and heavy-duty canvas duck slacks are found only in men's sizes. After a strenuous day of hiking, fishing, or hunting, a fatigued outdoor woman can have difficulty feeling feminine. But especially when she is dressed in baggy, shapeless, oversized pants, boots, shirts, and jacket.

At certain moments, every woodswoman has despaired of retaining femininity under mounds of men's clothing. Yet each has devised a secret formula that rejuvenates her spirit, refreshes femininity, and makes it glow. Marlene Simons (see Chapter 3), a big game hunting guide in northeastern Wyoming, suggests, "There are tricks to staying feminine in a man's world and one of mine is my small bottle of stick perfume (L'amiant by Cody). I keep it in my pocket. The men call it my buck scent because I am very lucky at seeing the good bucks and getting fellows shots when they are with me. Even outdoors you can remain a gal but being a good hunter and a fair shot doesn't just belong in a man's world."

Jane Baldwin packs a tube of Sweet Clover hand cream in her pack. "Hands really get rough and chapped while camping. I like the fragrance of Sweet Clover—clean and natural—and it attracts bees. They keep me company in the back country."

The taste, aroma, and moist sensation of freshly applied lipstick can spark newfound femininity in a woman within seconds. Or an outdoorswoman with pierced ears can feel her best when wearing a pair of conservative earrings. A mere touch of the hand to one earring can bolster sagging confidence. Perhaps a brisk brushing of the hair, stimulating circulation in the scalp, can rub away the shroud of exhaustion.

Some women prefer scarfs to hats. Tied peasant-style, a bright red bandana holds hair back out of the eyes, even on the windiest of days, and readily identifies one as feminine. On a scorching afternoon, this same scarf, dampened in a nearby stream, can dab refreshing coolness on the nape of the neck and all over the body. Or the wetted bandana,

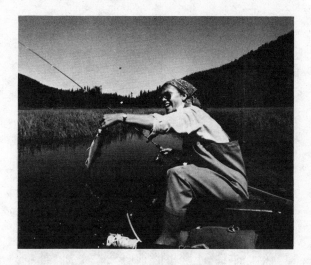

Femininity is how a woman sees herself. When wearing manly waders, a scarf can add a feminine touch.

tied around the forehead Indianlike, can soothe a hot brow and serve as a sweatband.

Bring a pair of sandals and shorts along. While impractical on the trail, at camp they bring out the woman in you. Shed the heavy hiking boots and wool socks. Slip on the sandals. Wiggle toes in the sand, test the water with the big toe and scamper through the dew. A pair of shorts can remind your companion, "Yes, indeed, you are woman." On a warm, bright day, you may want to nurture a tan. Then, a swim suit can express your femininity. In a cold mountain lake, a quick dunking in the icy water may be all you can tolerate. But, in warmer climates, a swim is a beautiful way to begin and end each day.

The trick to retaining femininity afield is first to know, wear, and bring along appropriate clothes and gear, yet, in addition, include something extra that makes you look

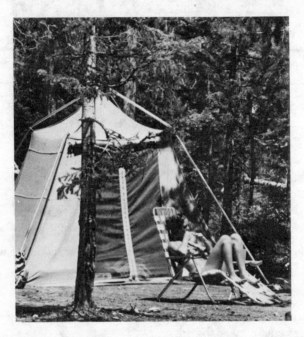

On a warm, bright day, a bikini can express your femininity.

or feel appealing, seductive, or refreshed. Exhaustion and fatigue are bound to hit an outdoorswoman at one time or another. At that moment, use your secret weapon.

DISCRIMINATION AGAINST OUTDOORSWOMEN

There is a great deal of talk about discrimination today. Joan Cone (see Chapter 1) believes outdoorswomen are subject to discrimination by sportsmen's groups and outdoor clothing manufacturers. In her opinion, one solution is for women to organize in a national outdoor women's association and lobby for changes. For further information, write to Outdoor Women, 500 Twelfth Street, S.W., Suite 810, Washington, D.C. 20024.

Joan is not alone. Of the twenty professional outdoorswomen interviewed, eight have experienced discrimination, eight have not, and four refused to answer the question. Significantly, three of the four who would not respond to the question occupy management positions in the National Park Service. The fourth is a resource assistant of the Forest Service. As she puts it, "I do not like to publicly discuss my personal feelings about working in a predominantly male field. Your questions seem to put me into a separate category from my fellow workers in that I may be breaking into a field where I have to fight to maintain my position because of my sex. There are some problems, I'll admit, but their causes are complex and are not necessarily generated from the fact that I am a woman. There have been occasions where being a female was a disadvantage as well as an advantage. I have tried to downplay this so it would not affect my job performance."

Two superintendents of National Historical Sites in California and one chief of an Archeological Center in Arizona refused to answer questions. All three basically said, "Since I do not feel that I am, in any way, an authority on the outdoors, I must defer. . . . While I have worked a number of years for the National Park Service, my career advancement has been in the field of management." These women, the heads of their respective National Park sites, apparently feel discriminated against to the point of not wanting to talk about it. They are defensive about being female and uncomfortable about being reminded of the fact.

Even though the Park Service allowed Jane Baldwin to participate in a rescue, women on the management level seem squeezed and threatened by the tenuous positions they hold.

On the other side of the discrimination barrier stands Dorothy Pilley as steadfast and strong as the mighty Alps that she loves. She began climbing mountains in the 1910s. Her book *Climbing Days* (Secker & Warburg, Ltd., 1935, 1965) records a personal, emotional account of twenty years of mountain climbing from northern Wales to the Alps, from the Rockies to the Himalayas. From friends she learned the techniques of mountaineering. She climbed extensively on her own and led groups along routes that she herself had discovered. She met and later married Professor I. A. Richards on a mountaineering expedition. Together they traveled and contested the world's giant peaks. Social restrictions influenced her to wear a skirt over tweed knicker-bockers until she reached the foot of the mountain. There she took off the skirt and cached it in a sack. Later, after the climb, she put the skirt back on to return to the city dressed in a respectable manner. In the 1890s, one of Dorothy's predecessors was Lucy Walker, the second president of the Ladies' Alpine Club. She always wore a red petticoat when climbing so that she could be easily found if she fell—and to conform to accepted feminine dress.

These women were true pioneers of the sport of mountaineering and of delineating women's place in the outdoors. The social declaration that ladies should always be seen in public wearing a skirt did not deter them. Such dictates were unimportant and petty to them. Their passion for mountain climbing was the central issue in their life. Everything else was secondary.

And then there is Georgie Clark. In the 1930s, she traveled west on a bicycle from Chicago to California. She was looking for adventure and a better life. During World War II, Georgie stumbled across the Colorado River. In the summers of 1945 and 1946, she swam 186 miles of the lower Colorado, learning about it firsthand. She has been on the river ever since.

In 1953 and 1954, she guided six people through the Grand Canyon on an Army surplus ten-person raft with one pair of oars. She invented the practice of tying together three ten-person rafts, which enabled the party to run the rapids instead of portaging around them. Instead of confronting the rapids straight on, she turned the craft broadside, giving it additional stability. Eventually she customized larger rafts and propelled them with motors up to twenty horsepower.

"As I look back over the wonderful years I have spent

outdoors—the largest percentage in connection with the Grand Canyon of the Colorado River—I feel that I have indeed been fortunate to miss out on discrimination. I was too far ahead of the gang to experience it. I have felt no discrimination, as such. In fact, I have had men ask me questions as to equipment and methods of solving various river problems. If my femininity has suffered there certainly has been no indication of it from the men.

"I have always wanted to be out-of-doors and let very little stand in my way insofar as being there. When I first viewed the Colorado River, I knew it was to be my hobby— one way or another—for the rest of my life, if my wonderful health stood up. Well, it did and the river really became a hobby. I hiked it, swam it, rowed it and traversed it in every kind of boat I could get my hands on. When concessions became available, I saw an opportunity to make a wonderful hobby pay me something in return and it is proving that way. I certainly have no complaints.

"There was no competition. I was not compared to any one. I felt no need to defend any of my trials and errors— being tough-skinned or defensive would only have made my goal harder to reach. I learned to back up and start over if I met a problem that looked too big at the moment.

"I have always felt that a Grand Canyon Experience is most desirable for the person who appreciates the outdoors, and it was with this thought in mind that I continued to search for ways to have more companions on the river with me. That thought mothered the idea of tying the boats together to make a large raft. After that, the river became a water highway. I had plenty of company on my trips but the competition with other outfitters became a big factor.

"I believe any woman can enter the outdoor field and accomplish anything she sets her mind on. She does have to be realistic in so far as health is concerned. She has to work at it, be determined and know that she is going to have to earn her own way. She will accomplish just as much as she puts into it."

Strong-willed, bold, autonomous, Georgie is a legend to everyone who has been bounced, whipped, bruised by the violent, merciless yet entrancing Colorado.

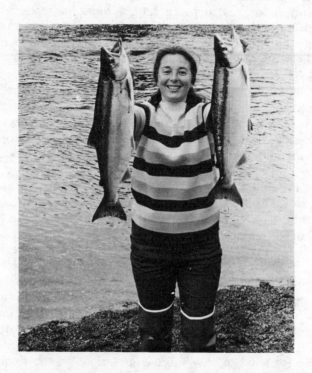

Even on the Situk River in Alaska, holding two mammoth sockeye salmon she has just caught, Peggy Bauer is the picture of femininity.—*Photo by Erwin A. Bauer*

As Peggy Bauer (see Chapter 1) sums it up, "Femininity is an asset. Retaining it is like considering whether to have brown eyes. There they are and there they will stay and it's all part of the whole. It wasn't femininity that got in the way in the early part of my adulthood. It was the pervasive opinion that women, even well-educated women, got married to a rising young corporate executive; kept a dust-free home; and had a large family of well-adjusted children, who never felt a twinge of sibling rivalry."

Femininity is learned and yet each woman adds a unique touch to the concept. Each woman is female and yet she expresses her gender in a special way. Nature can help her be even more womanly by offering new ways of expression as well as inspiring more ideas to communicate. Nature can bring out the best in a woman but not unless the woman feels her best. That is, be willing to accept the challenge. Yes, discrimination can exist for the outdoorswoman but the most effective way to combat it, render it impotent, is to go out into the wilderness alone.

Follow your interests. Let your fancy be your guide. Whether the direction be the river, woods, mountain, field, sky, ocean, when you enter the new scene, it will no longer be the same and neither will you. You will be more—much more—of a woman.

5

Outdoor Comfort

Rain pounds earthlings. Gray gauze clouds descend upon the landscape. Reach out and touch the foggy shroud. Unable to see beyond a foot or two, you sit transfixed within the opaque stillness of a carbonated soda bubble. Clouds nozzle droplets with driving force to penetrate the thirsty ground and saturate living creatures.

Buttercups glisten. Harebells droop. Magpies ruffle moist feathers. Streams swell. Trails liquify. Cottonwoods drip. The air shivers and overflows with dampness. The world is wet but you are dry, warm, and fascinated by the fresh, clean, renewing effect of a hard, thorough rain.

You feel good. Raingear enables you to wander into the heart of the cloudburst without fear of being damp and cold. Attention is directed outward to the surrounding sights, sounds, and heady smells. The spirit of exploration takes over. You become infatuated with the small, soggy world. Walking in the rain unconcerned frees the civilized mind. The downpour tingles the skin and rolls off your shoulders just as it does from a duck's back. Bad weather no longer dominates you. Venture into nature regardless of rain, wind, snow. You are alive, refreshing, and attractive. Concerns leave. What remains is your soul, the core, simply you. You look great.

How can this be? How can a person learn to enjoy bad weather? The secret is the way you dress. Foul weather clothes form a protective layer between you and the environment. Let it rain. Your body maintains a constant, comfortable temperature. Snowflakes, peanut-size hail, and raindrops cannot permeate either clothing or your spirit. Bad weather apparel is like a vaccination. You are immunized. Pursue the novelties of the outdoors oblivious to its changing, sometimes drizzly moods.

With bad weather gear, a camper will not be hampered by outside forces. She actually welcomes dark foreboding skies, rumblings, and occasional lightning as part of the wilderness scene. Knowledge, practice, and a capsule of common sense are necessary to thrive in any type of weather. But it is possible. In fact, it is fundamental to a satisfying, stable relationship with the outdoors. The woodswoman needs to know how to handle sudden outbursts from sometimes temperamental nature.

Feeling good in the outdoors begins with being warm and dry. Do not depend on a campfire for heat or on a shelter, such as a tent, for protection from rain or snow. Even though these can supplement comfort in the wilderness during bad weather, a camper can dress to safeguard body and spirit against the dampening, chilling effect of two weeks of thundersqualls.

THE LAYER SYSTEM OF WEARING CLOTHING

Wear layers of clothes. Lightweight, summery items, like a halter, short-sleeve or thin cotton blouse, are worn as the first layer, next to the skin. Then, a flannel or wool shirt or sweater, followed by a goose down vest or heavy jacket and topped off with a waterproof windbreaker. This series of layers will protect the torso against any type of weather.

As afternoon approaches and temperature rises, gradually peel off the outside layers until you feel comfortable. Begin the shedding process, or "ventilation," as soon as you be-

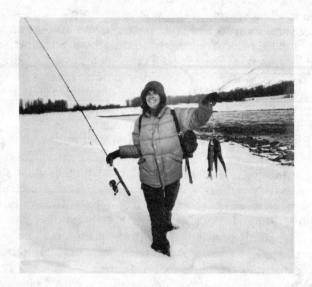

Wear layers of clothes for warmth and comfort in any kind of weather.

come hot. This cools the body and prevents the garments
next to the skin from absorbing perspiration. Once cotton
becomes saturated with perspiration, body heat is drawn
away and wasted in an attempt to warm up the wet clothes.
As a result, chill can take over, producing clamminess and
misery.

Pack the extra garments into a day pack or backpack.
Later, when temperatures drop, replace the layers. In this
way, a person can achieve warmth or coolness by degrees.
The combination of clothes can meet nearly any kind of
atmospheric condition.

Choose camping clothes according to warmth, comfort
and protection. Roomy rather than snug-fitting, they should
be made of cotton or wool. Even though synthetic fabrics
are comfortable at home or office, they offer little warmth
and protection. Wind breezes right through the porous

structure of polyesters and insects can bite through them as well. Dress as if you expect the worst possible weather—that is, in the mountains expect wind and snow; predict rain in the lowlands and scorching temperatures in the desert.

Practicality governs what to wear outdoors. Forget fashion and fads. Shorts and sandals are meant for the smooth, briarless, level cement sidewalks of the city. They fail to protect the skin. On the contrary, they leave too much of the body exposed and vulnerable. Thorned

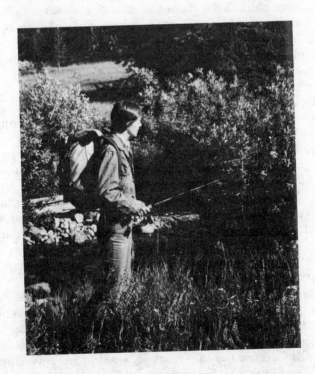

When temperature rises, peel off the outside layers of clothes and pack them away in a day pack.

berry bushes and mosquitoes are attracted to sweet, uncovered flesh.

COLD WEATHER CLOTHING

In snow or where temperatures drop below forty degrees, wool is the best fabric to wear. It warms and protects the body better than any other material. Wool is tightly woven and guards against insect bites as well as scratches from tree limbs and brush. A pair of wool slacks enables you to walk through heavy vegetation without a scrape or sit on a crusted snowbank without getting wet.

Wool "breathes." It allows air to pass back and forth through the fibers. Air cools and evaporates moisture forming on the skin. This prevents excessive sweating. In the mountains, wool hiking pants can be beneficial even during June, July, and August.

Wool shirts retain body heat and produce a cocoon sense of security. A shirt that buttons down the front is practical. When too warm, unbutton the shirt, letting more air inside to circulate. The opening down the front offers another layer of cooling or warmth without actually removing or adding an article of clothing.

Wool socks prevent blisters and entrapment of perspiration. By wearing two pairs, the feet are encapsulated against the cold and abrasions.

Wool gloves insulate fingers and hands against biting frost. Fingers generally serve as the body's thermometer and are first to experience a drop in temperature. Inactive hands can be numbed by frigid weather in a matter of minutes. At high elevations, wool gloves may be required throughout most of the year.

A wool stocking cap shields ears, head and face from severe weather. Low nighttime temperatures may require a camper to wear one while sleeping. A wool cap assists in keeping body heat inside the sleeping bag. In this way, it forestalls "sleeping cold"—that is, waking up shivering. A wool head covering redirects body heat down around the body and counteracts warmth escaping through the bag opening. Instead of vainly trying to sleep while chilled, the camper rests soundly.

Long Underwear

Long underwear is a woodswoman's second layer of skin. It traps body heat and holds it close to the body for added warmth. In this way, body heat is recycled, so to speak, and not lost to cold weather. Thus, long underwear serves well as a set of pajamas.

On warmer days or during strenuous exercise, excessive perspiration is absorbed by long underwear, which becomes wet and clammy. Once long underwear is damp, it becomes a detriment, ultimately inflicting chills unless removed and dried.

Duofold is a brand name of long underwear that consists of two layers of material: a cotton layer for comfort and a wool one for warmth and ventilation. Between the two layers, an air space acts as an insulator. This type of underwear is effective if the camper does not perspire heavily. Once saturated, it too becomes useless.

Fishnet long underwear is best for persons who perspire freely or for those who plan on strenuous activity, such as mountain climbing. Net underwear is made of cotton or a wool-cotton blend with plenty of circulation holes in it, thus resembling a fishnet. In cold weather, body heat is trapped and retained in the open mesh air pockets between the skin and the next layer of clothing. At higher temperatures, the netted weave facilitates air circulation necessary to prevent clothes from being soaked with perspiration. Woolen fishnet is more expensive but more effective than cotton.

Down- or polyester-insulated long underwear is too hot for most active outdoorswomen unless they are snowmobiling or ice fishing where there is never enough warmth. A moderate level of activity results in heavy perspiring with such a thick layer of insulation next to the skin. However, some women sleep in it or use it as loungewear around camp. It nearly guarantees warmth in the sleeping bag or around the campfire.

Underwear made of virgin wool is the best heat stimulator. But wool is not as comfortable (it scratches) as cotton and costs twice as much. Wool long underwear would be practical for very cold winters and for hunters who sit in duck or goose blinds in zero-degree or below temperatures.

Gaiters

Gaiters are nylon leggings that prevent snow from entering the boot and safeguard the foot and lower leg from icy wetness. They normally extend from the foot over the boot to below the knee. Snowshoers, skiers, hunters, and ice fisherwomen recognize the usefulness of gaiters. They can be purchased from sporting goods stores, ski shops, or mail-order companies such as Eddie Bauer (Seattle, Wash.), L. L. Bean (Freeport, Maine), or Paul Petzoldt Wilderness Equipment (Lander, Wyo.).

Gaiters are easy to design and sew yourself once a finished pair has been examined. The hardest step is finding suitable material. Use coated nylon for the outside layer and uncoated nylon as the inside layer. Avoid elastic on gaiters because it tends to cut off circulation in the leg or ankle. Instead, employ drawstrings to secure the gaiter to the boot as well as to tie the top part around the calf. A plastic YKK zipper facilitates putting on and removing. However, cover the zipper with a flap of material so snow and ice will not ooze through the zipper teeth and saturate the leg.

RAINGEAR

Nylon jacket and pants and wide-brimmed hat form the waterproof shield that enables a camper to walk carefree in wind and rain. Sporting goods stores and mail-order warehouses offer a wide variety of raingear.

Foul weather apparel should be roomy to fit over several layers of clothes. Construction is important. Water soaks through seams and other types of stitching. Check that these vulnerable spots are double-stitched and protected with flaps where needed.

Rain Jacket and Pants

For hikers, campers, fisherwomen, and hunters who are on the move and have limited packing space, lightweight raingear is perfect. Weighing less than sixteen ounces, rain jacket and pants can be folded small enough to fit into a pocket. Stored in a fishing vest or a day pack, they are within easy reach to put on at the first splash of a raindrop or gust of wind.

The big question in choosing the right raingear for you is: of what type of nylon is it made? The fabric of most bad weather clothes is nylon, coated with polyurethane. Even though the coating repels water from the outside environment, it tends to cause a buildup of moisture on the inside from perspiration and condensation. The reason? Polyurethane robs nylon of its ability to breathe. That is, air can no longer circulate through the nylon fibers once they are coated. Ironically, although a coated nylon jacket and pair of pants can protect the clothes from wind and rain, they act as a steambath to the body. Moisture accumulates on the skin surface, dampening the clothes, which produces chilling.

Nylon taffeta is usually not coated. As a result, it breathes, allowing fresh air through the fabric weave to cool off the body. However, it is not completely waterproof. While the bulk of the rain rolls off taffeta, a degree of moisture soaks into the material. This phenomenon is not serious if the hiker has followed the layered principle of dressing. Then, there are several layers between the wet rain jacket and the body. This situation is more healthy than having droplets accumulate inside as happens with coated nylon raingear.

Many times, the label on foul weather gear does not specify whether the material is coated. In this case, test it yourself. Put a section of the jacket or pants to your lips. Breathe in through your mouth. If air does not flow through the nylon into your mouth, the fabric is coated. If air travels through the material, it is uncoated and breathes.

Effective bad weather gear is expensive. Pants average about $18; jackets, approximately $23 to $27. Nylon is sold in fabric stores by the yard, and certain patterns can be altered to make rain pants and jacket at home. Be sure to attach a hood on the jacket and to put elastic where you normally would put hooks, snaps, or buttons. Velcro strips can replace zippers, which can be weak spots where rain seeps in.

Cagoule

A cagoule is an elongated hooded rain parka that extends below the knees. It keeps the entire body dry, eliminating the need for rain pants. In emergency situations, with the hood over the head, it can also serve as a makeshift tent. While the cagoule sounds versatile and useful, it can be a nuisance. It is bulky and interferes with brisk hiking. Even though it has a drawstring around the bottom to tie around the waist when the full length is not needed, it drops down easily. The cagoule gets entangled in heavy underbrush. And it can become hooked around the saddle while you are riding a horse. As a result, dismounting is awkward.

Poncho

A poncho is a rectangular section of coated nylon with a slot in the middle for your head. It hangs loosely over the entire body and sheds rain. Because it is not secured to the body, except by sleeve snaps, it promotes air circulation and prevents condensation on the inside of the poncho. However, this feature can be a serious detriment on gusty, rainy days. The wind flares the poncho, rendering it virtually useless to ward off the effects of rain. In addition, a poncho can be dangerous to a campfire cook. The wind could easily blow a corner of the poncho into the fire. Caution should be exercised by the poncho wearer around a flame.

PROTECTION FROM THE SUN

A wide-brimmed hat, sunglasses, a long-sleeved cotton blouse, and heavy-duty cotton slacks are the best defense against intense sun. Carry plenty of fluids and ingest salt tablets or salt dissolved in water. An alternative to salt is instant Gatorade. Mix with water and drink. It relieves thirst as well as meets the salt requirement.

When desert camping, bring along a wool shirt and warm sleeping bag for the typically cool nights. Siesta instead of travel during the heat of the day. Seek or build shade during high noon (11 A.M. until 3 P.M.). Hike in the morning or towards evening but before dark. To avoid blistering sunburn, dab sunscreen lotion on exposed skin, including hands, nose, forehead, ears.

Compared to the other types of foul weather, sun can be the most deadly. Yes, sun. Worshipers of *el sol* fail to realize that heat stroke, heat exhaustion, and burn shock may result from overexposure to infrared and ultraviolet rays on a hot humid day anywhere in the United States. But by using common sense, keeping the body covered, and resting in the shade when tired, the outdoorswoman can avoid the ill effects of overexposure to the sun.

HOW TO VENT YOUR FRUSTRATIONS

When a woodswoman makes a mistake in the backcountry, the results hover over her longer than they would at home. She forgot to pack the raingear before leaving camp and walking two miles to a golden trout pond. Then, it began to rain. Now, warming over a fire, she is wet, mad at herself, and miserable. This condition will continue until next morning, when she is rested, dry, and anticipating a new day.

But there is a way to vent anger, disappointment, or other negative feelings when alone in the backwoods. Write them down. A $.35 notebook, small enough to fit into the pocket of a pair of jeans, can be the means to feeling good once again after a frustrating ordeal. Even while you are recording the incident on paper, the humor hits you. The comedy of errors. How you must have looked! If only your friends could have seen you!

Besides being an emotional release, a daily log records the details of the trip. Little things that you will want to remember at a later date but will likely slip your mind. What fly did I catch those golden trout on? What kind of berry did I identify near the lake? What dehydrated dish was so delicious?

By rereading your ups and downs, discoveries and challenges, you relive the excitement, the adventure of the backpack hike.

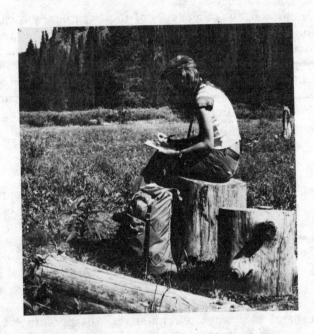

Log experiences in a notebook both as an emotional release and an accurate record of your trip.

BEING PREPARED FOR EMERGENCIES

While packing for an extended trip into the wilderness (longer than one week), think of items that are hard to do without and that would assist with an aggravating predicament. What if the tent ripped? Pack a needle and a spool of thread. What would happen if a button from your slacks popped? Bring several safety pins.

How do you find your way in the dark? Include a flashlight. How miserable if your hiking boots rubbed blisters on the heel of your foot. Store a tube of medicated cream and a supply of band-aids in the side pocket of your pack. Maybe your fingernail will break off, leaving a jagged edge. Slip an emory board in with the provisions.

These articles are practical remedies for bothersome dilemmas. Without them, the trouble would linger until you returned home.

Some outdoorswomen would not venture afield without a container of vitamins. Each morning they take a vitamin for necessary nourishment to sustain a rugged pace. Even though dehydrated and freeze-dried food contains vitamins, meals in the outdoors can be irregular. When considering the fatigue that incapacitates the woman who does not eat properly, the price of vitamins is inexpensive. They are insurance that the body is in top condition nutritionally.

INSECT REPELLENTS

Insect bites and stings and poison ivy, oak, and sumac can be problems in the wilds. Old-timers smeared mud on exposed flesh to discourage flies, mosquitoes, ticks, and chiggers. Today scientists report that citronella oil is the number one natural insect repellent. One study reported that vitamin B-1 taken in large doses (50 mg/day for the week prior to the trip and 10 mg twice a day during the outing) produces an odor through the skin of the individual that drives mosquitoes off. Eating lots of garlic is another weapon against pesky insects.

The effectiveness of commercially produced insect repellent seems to vary from one location to another. Upon arriving in a new town, inquire about the favorite bug lotion. Otherwise, test the leading repellents yourself: Muskol, Off, Cutter's and Mosquitone. Cigar smoke assists these brands in building a protective barrier that insects find hard to penetrate. A lady *should* accept a Tiparillo.

POISONOUS PLANTS

Recognizing and avoiding poison ivy, oak, and sumac are the recommended ways of dealing with these plants. If you suspect you have come in contact with them, wash yourself and clothes with a strong soap. This will cut down

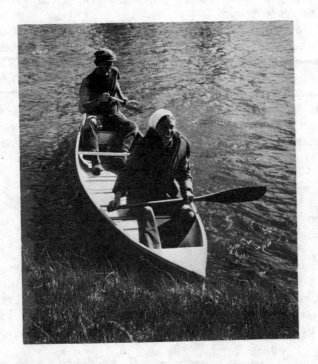

When you feel good, you look even better.

the "poison" and wash it harmlessly away. In addition, massive doses (1 gram/day or 1000 mg/day) of Vitamin C have allegedly lowered sensitivity to poison ivy. Even so, train your eye to spot and shun the rash-producing plants. Plant identification books can help.

Nature has a few rough edges. You can dress, pack, and learn to smooth them out into harmless challenges. But this demands thought, preparation, and common sense. As a result, you feel good and look even better. You cannot help being feminine. As Lynn Thomas, a writer and inventor living in San Francisco, puts it, "I think it is extremely important to retain my femininity. But that implies that I must work to retain it. And I do not. It is an integral part of my being. . . . Men who backpack treat me like a princess. They fall in love with me—at least for a little while—because men seek female companionship on the trail, and their women don't backpack." And if you feel like a princess, you are bound to act like one.

6

Camping Skills

A naiad is a nymph who gives life to springs, fountains, rivers, and lakes and who inhabits the environment she has created. This fair mythological maiden was believed responsible for the allure and the soothing, entrancing effect of a woodland pond on the human spirit. But, alas, her possessive charm had the potentially destructive power of holding an enchanted man breathless beneath her surface, ultimately drowning him.

The modern woman finds herself in much the same dilemma as the naiad of old. Whether she realizes it or not, she designs and constructs her own environment as well as her position there. She can be a meek, mild servant of a large family, an aggressive, bold leader of a professional group, or someone in between these extremes. The choice is hers. Unfortunately, the mechanics of building her life's atmosphere generally occurs during early adulthood or late adolescence when the meaning of life and the significance of her role have not yet reached consciousness. Too often, the fibers of her style are woven haphazardly, even blindly, resulting in a jumbled, uncoordinated tapestry. As a result, years go by while she passively watches her surroundings turn a murky blah color as if the entire system were out of control, beyond her limited influence.

But this is far afield from the truth. Femininity does not exclude independence and self-sufficiency. On the contrary, the more spunky the woman, the more men (and women) want to be around her.

A spirited, action-oriented person develops through years of achievement. As a youth, athletic skills are important. Adequate physical education can teach a youngster poise and confidence as well as the mechanics of a sport and the benefits of physical fitness. But such training for girls is often overlooked.

Micki King is the recognized leader of those who are working for the amateur athlete's rights. In the 1972 Olympics in Munich, Germany, Micki won the gold medal in the three-meter springboard diving competition. Now a captain in the Air Force and a full-time physical education instructor at the Air Force Academy, Micki believes that women should organize and strive for appropriate recognition and the chance to develop athletically. "Basically the same problems exist in women's athletics as exist for women in all fields. Equal opportunity is the key."

A recent federal law stipulates that educational institutions receiving federal funds must provide equal opportunity in all programs for both men and women. Including athletics.

However, the physical education of boys and girls, men and women, should not stop with fitness programs and competition. Physical education should expand into the outdoor realm where students learn how to handle themselves in the backcountry. How to choose a campsite and set up a comfortable home base. How to build a fire—even in the rain—and to cook succulent, nourishing meals over its searing coals. Physical education should teach about the outdoors and help an individual practice what she has learned. The daily demands of the wilds call for a physical yet knowledgeable response. Backwoods skills inspire self-sufficiency not only in the wilderness but among other humans. Enjoy and live with nature. Through a combination of physical fitness, stamina, and dexterity, create your own niche outdoors.

CHOOSING A CAMPSITE

A campsite is where you will spend one or more nights outdoors. Even though there are limitless possibilities, there are certain features that make one campsite better than another.

In organized campgrounds, find a spot that is a convenient distance from the bathhouse yet not next door to it. It should have at least one large tree or bush to provide shade and protection from wind or rain. A ready supply of firewood is a bonus. Often the scarcity of deadfall may require the camper to buy firewood from a vendor. It should be separated from nearby campsites by trees and bushes, giving the impression you are isolated from civilization, even if you are surrounded by other tenters. But most importantly, there should be a level portion of ground where you can pitch your tent or park your camper.

Many "campgrounds" that offer hookups (electricity, water and sewage unit) closely resemble parking lots. With no other alternative, you must accept the situation. However, careful planning on a camping vacation can direct you to Orange Grove Campgrounds in the South, for instance, where orange trees bearing fruit separate one campsite from the next. Through the tent window, reach out and pick a blazing, juicy orange for breakfast.

In the backwoods, where camping at a designated campsite is not necessary, choosing a camping locale is a challenge. Look for one near a stream or spring where fresh, drinkable water is obtainable. Within ten feet from a large, protective tree or bush, a level spot with an abundance of deadfall timber for a campfire is ideal.

Because the campsite will be home for awhile, select one that appeals to you. Stretch out on the ground a minute and test the slope of the area. Even though it might appear level, a gradual incline can disturb restful sleep. The choice is personal. Does the location offer a promise of fantastic

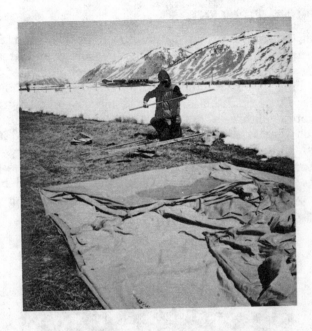

Choose a campsite that is level, free of rocks and snow, and that appeals to you.

fishing, wild flower hunting or photography? Then, settle there.

Begin the campsite search early in the day. In the organized campgrounds of popular national parks, such as the Grand Canyon, campsites are commonly all occupied on a first-come, first-served basis by 10 A.M. While camping in more remote areas, 3:00 P.M. is about the right time to locate a campsite. Set up camp with fire blazing and begin dinner around dusk. Avoid waiting until dark to do camp chores. Without the accustomed electric lights, the outdoors is darker than black. Each simple task requires extra concentration and effort. You can lose your way while trying to find water and firewood. The night is for star-gazing, storytelling, and sleep—not for work.

PITCHING THE TENT

Setting up camp is primarily a matter of organization. Pitch the tent on a flat, rock-free piece of ground and arrange the rest of the gear within convenient reach.

Pitching a tent is much like putting together a jigsaw puzzle. First, read the directions. Then, by following each step, abracadabra, a tent stands taut and cozy before you.

Each tent is different with a personality and idiosyncrasies. Initially, a new tent may take as long as thirty minutes to assemble. But, with subsequent pitchings, the time lessens and the ease increases until the experienced backwoodswoman can put a tent together in five or ten minutes.

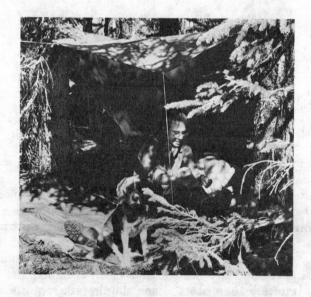

On short trips during good weather, a tarp can replace a tent.

On short trips during good weather, a camper can substitute a tarp and a section of nylon rope for a tent. Tarps are commonly made of ripstop nylon, coated with urethane or other waterproofing agent. A large tarp (ten feet square) weighs about three pounds and costs approximately $25. Compared to the price of tents, ($60 and up), tarps cannot be beat. They afford protection from sun, rain, and snow. However, they are not efficient in high wind.

Along the sides of a tarp are metal grommets or tie tabs. The camper ties nylon rope to the grommets, stretches the tarp into a protective covering, and secures the other end of the rope to tree or rock anchors. A small primitive pup tent can be made from a tarp. First, string a rope between two trees, about three feet above the ground. Drape the tarp over the rope and stake the corners to the earth. Or a lean-to can be constructed by tying two corners to a tree and staking the other side to the ground. With a lighted match, ignite the end of the nylon rope for a minute to melt the tip and prevent unraveling.

A tarp is the closest thing to "sleeping under the stars," yet having a degree of protection from rain and dew. But for long periods of bad weather, only a tent can keep the camper warm, dry, and comfortable.

Tarps are versatile. Use one as a ground cloth to protect the sleeping bag from moisture and punctures. Or spread over the woodpile during a thunderstorm to keep the wood dry, crisp, and ready. A space blanket makes an excellent makeshift tarp.

Some sporting goods stores rent tents. Try several different makes and models and decide for yourself the one that is best for you. For a woman, the backpack tent is usually simpler, easier to set up, and lighter than larger ones. A backpack tent is made of uncoated nylon to prevent condensation developing on the inside wall and ceiling. It generally weighs from four to six pounds, including tent pegs and poles. To waterproof the tent, a rain fly is necessary. This is a piece of coated nylon or canvas that covers only the top of the tent. To top off the tent with a rain fly involves a little extra effort but is invaluable when a sudden shower strikes.

Nylon coverings and screens for tent windows and doors are recommended. Strong, durable, easy to manage zippers usually distinguish the top-quality tent from the mediocre.

Pegs are an integral part of all tents. Hammer tent pegs into the ground through loops on the outside of the tent floor. Depending on the type of soil, this can be an easy or difficult task. Rocky soil, common in the mountains, is difficult to penetrate. Sandy soil as found in the Southwest, may not hold the peg securely. A large rock can be used as a hammer. If you are willing to carry the extra weight, a hatchet in a sheath, attached to your belt, is a handy camping tool. It serves as a hammer to pound in tent pegs and can double as a saw to chop firewood.

A backpack tent is small like a pup tent. You can sit upright in one but not stand. However, it is wide and long enough to sleep two cozily with room left over to store gear. Consider tents that feature an aluminum or fiberglass pole frame, designed to structure the tent from the outside. Poles that brace the tent from the inside for stability greatly reduce roominess.

In addition, veer away from tents that require "guy ropes." A guy rope extends from the tent and must be tied to pegs hammered into the ground several feet away from the tent. Guy ropes stretch the sides of the tent tight and smooth without wrinkles. In turn, this improves the stability and weather resistance of the tent. On the other hand, a tent with guy ropes takes about twice as long to set up. Beware of the guys: they are booby traps that trip. While they may be required on mountaineering expeditions or heavy-duty winter camping, they are merely troublesome for the average camper.

If you prefer the added room and convenience of a full-size tent (8 feet by 10 feet or bigger), there is an endless variety. Again, these large tents, whether canvas or nylon, require a rain fly as waterproof protection. An eight-by-ten tent serves two adults or a family of four in comfortable style. The camper can stand erect with room to spare and can even cook inside during foul weather. However, it is more complicated and time-consuming to assemble.

A pop-up tent is full-size, usually made of a canvas-duck

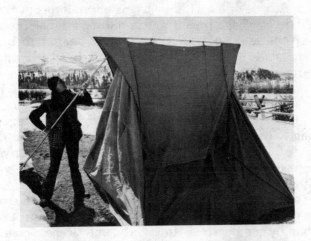

After a few practice runs, this 8 x 10 canvas tent is easy for a woman alone to set up.

material. Its bonus is ease in setting up. After putting the outside frame of poles together, the tent "pops up" and can be moved without disassembling short distances. Raising this tent requires the coordinated effort of two campers. A woman alone would have difficulty pitching it.

Become proficient in erecting your tent in the backyard before entering the wilderness. Once you get the knack, you will never forget. You—pitching a tent. Can you imagine?

FURNISHING THE TENT

Once the tent is erected—facing the most picturesque direction—furnish it with camping gear. Transform it into a home. Put the foam pad or cot on the floor; pull the sleeping bag from its storage sack and fluff it up. Place the pillow at the head (or, on a backpack trip, stuff the sleeping bag sack with extra clothes for a makeshift pillow). The downy cocoon beckons you to lie a minute and test its seductive comfort. But, no, there is much more to do.

Stash extra clothes within easy reach underneath the cot or next to the bag. Insects and moisture are not problems because the tent floor acts as a barrier against them. Arrange toiletries in an out-of-the-way place to avoid rummaging through the car or pack.

A number of campers use sleeping bag liners. A liner, commonly made of soft, washable flannel, is as long and wide as the bag. Its main function is to absorb dirt and keep the bag soil-free. Each washing or dry cleaning of a down or Dacron Fiberfill II bag reduces the loft and effectiveness to a certain degree. The liner lessens the need for frequent cleaning.

In colder climates, the liner is insulated with Dacron or prime goose down which in turn increases the comfort range of a bag by ten degrees. However, some sleepers complain that the liner is too confining and inhibiting.

Cooking and Eating Equipment

Down home cooking and mouth-watering eating revolve around a reliable, easy-to-regulate heat source. Sometimes it is impractical or against campground rules to build a fire. For this reason, it is smart to pack along a cook stove.

Outdoor Stoves. An outdoor stove can have one, two, or three burners, fueled by propane, butane, white gas, kerosene, or alcohol. The type and size of the stove depend on the individual needs of the camper. Backpack stoves, for instance, are single burners, fueled by white gas, kerosene, butane, or propane. Propane and white gas are the two most popular types of backpack fuels. Propane is economical, comes in refillable canisters, and cannot be spilled. In addition, it is lighter in weight and does not require priming or pumping as does white gas. Before purchasing a backpack stove, carefully consider the price against the weight and compactability of the stove. Every ounce and inch count in backpacking. Also, ease of operation and dependability under adverse weather conditions are essential.

For family or group camping from a vehicle where weight and space are insignificant, try a two- or three-burner stove. Outdoor cooking then is nearly as simple and easy as using the range at home. Again, white gas or propane are two standbys as fuel for larger cook stoves.

Consumer statistics report that the Coleman two-burner, white-gas stove is most popular among campers. Since 1923, the Coleman Company has been manufacturing camp stoves. In fact, its 1929 model is exactly like the one on the market today. This fact alone is testimony to its convenience and reliability. It folds up into a small suitcase-size package with a handle. White gas stoves need to be pumped and then lighted. But once you read and follow the directions, a little practice makes operation a cinch. The flame is regulated in the same manner as on a gas range.

A two- or three-burner stove can be elevated to a waist-high level by setting it on a collapsible metal-frame stand. This folds up into an elongated package, the size of a folded umbrella. No longer does the camp cook have to stoop to stir the stew or flip the pancakes. With the stove off the ground, the danger of insects invading the food is lessened.

Water Jug. Next to the stove, water is the most vital tool to the camp cook. It is the wise camper who packs a five-gallon jug (with spigot) of water in the back of her vehicle. Water vitalizes dehydrated and freeze-dried food into gourmet meals. Water refreshes aching muscles and sagging energy. Water washes away the grime of fatigue both inside and outside the body (see Chapter 7). Hang the jug or pouch of water near the stove on a tree limb or a large rock.

Pots and Pans. When selecting cooking equipment, follow the "can-do-without-if-I-need-to" principle. Even though camp can be a comfortable refuge, it need not be another home with all the luxuries. If you forget something, that makes the trip even more memorable. It is surprising—even mystifying—how humans can improvise when forced to. However, they refuse to practice this intriguing talent unless there is no other way out. A basic number of pots and pans is necessary of course, but do not attempt to include omelet pan, waffle iron, and electric can opener.

For the solitary camper, a skillet and a two-quart pot with lid are the only cooking artillery required. For a family or camping group of four, a four-quart pan and a kettle may be added. The secret of getting by with so few pots lies in careful preplanning of meals. The incidental cooking utensils are a wooden spoon, a spatula, lids for the pots, and removable handles or a pair of pliers for transferring steaming pans from one burner to another. Purchase pans that "nest"—that is, that fit one inside the other. Then, no matter how many pots you bring, they take up only as much room as the largest one. Interchangeable lids and handles are convenient.

If camping from a vehicle, a worthwhile substitute for the skillet is a griddle. Teflon-coated, it fits perfectly over a two-burner white-gas stove. On it, pancakes can be made for a crowd without sticking or fish can be fried whole without curling.

Plates, Cups, and Silverware. Eating gear too should fall in line with the plain-and-simple rule. Paper plates and cups, forks, and spoons are all that is needed. Paper napkins and towels are handy. Burn the used plates. This, in turn, keeps the cleaning chores to a minimum.

Place the cooking and eating equipment on or near the stove. By organizing the necessary tools in one location, the ordeal of searching will be eliminated. The most frustrating aspect of camp cooking is not knowing where everything is. By keeping gear close at hand, the cook can create without missing an ingredient.

Instant Food. When backpacking, the camper relies on instant food—dehydrated and freeze-dried meals and add-only-water drinks. Otherwise, cold canned drinks, steaks, chops, and sandwich fixings can be brought along. To do this, of course, a portable ice box—a cooler—is necessary.

Coolers. Coolers come in nearly as many sizes and shapes as campers do. Some, made of styrofoam, are inexpensive, but break down under heavy use. Others are sturdy, welded steel boxes with plenty of insulation that can last a sensible lifetime. The cooler should have a tight-lipped seal with a sturdy, dependable latch that bars insects, intense heat, severe cold, and other intruders.

A twenty-quart cooler with a ten-pound block of ice is unbeatable. It will defend perishables under the threat of boiling sun and a swarm of flies. Ice chests come smaller and larger. Shop around and decide which one will fit your needs. But, the bigger the chest, the more ice is needed. The total weight of a large cooler filled with ice and food might be muscle- and back-wrenching.

Nothing is more appreciated on a hot, dusty day of fishing or traveling than a frosty drink from an ice-cold cooler. But it needs special treatment. Keep it out of the sun and avoid opening the lid frequently. Each time the seal is broken, more ice disappears into liquid which in turn dissolves more of the precious frozen crystals. Place the cooler in the shade next to the tent. It will be there when you need it—and during the summer you will need it often.

BUILDING A FIRE

Fundamentally, a fire is a large flame that sustains itself and grows from a ready supply of fuel, usually dry wood. There is a lot of discussion about slow-burning versus fast-burning wood. Oak, for example, burns slowly while pine is consumed faster. A camper will use whatever wood is available regardless of its blazing speed. This is a matter of common sense.

A fire begins with a small flame produced by striking a match. Unless fed, the flame will die. For nourishment, it requires a diet of dry, old (that is, not green) wood. First, let the flame devour a small pile of "twiggies." Twiggies are the tiniest dead branches on the bottom trunk of trees and shrubs. Toothpick-size, without leaves or needles, they can be easily snapped off the tree with a twist of the wrist. A flame also readily eats up lichen (a type of dry moss) or

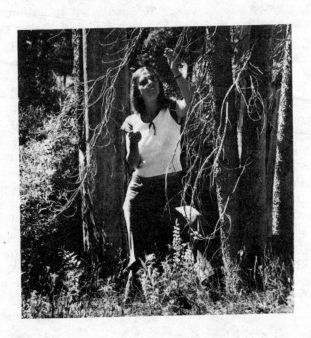

A campfire begins with a small pile of "twiggies," the tiny dead branches on the bottom of trees and shrubs.

brown pine needles and leaves. Once the flame has grown into a small fire by engulfing the pile of twiggies, put slightly bigger twigs and branches on it. Remember to give the fire plenty of breathing room until the flame is going strong. Many fires are smothered by putting on too much wood too soon. The bigger the fire, the larger branches it can swallow. However, a small fire demands smaller twigs. Otherwise, it will choke on the branches and die out. Break the twigs into six-inch lengths. Begin very small and grow with the flame.

Before striking the first match, gather the necessary wood. This procedure lends order to firemaking and relieves the fire builder from frantic searchings for wood while the small fire is smoldering. Three-inch-long wooden matches that can strike anywhere are ideal for campfires. They maintain a safe distance between flame and finger. In addition, they burn longer under the mound of twiggies than do cardboard or shorter matches, thus increasing the combustible time. A convenient spot for striking wooden matches is the zipper of your jeans or hiking slacks. This method is more dependable than trying to strike matches on a nearby, damp rock and the zipper is right there with you, near the pile of twiggies.

Build a fire away from a tree. Otherwise, dancing flames may ignite an overhanging limb. If there is no fireplace already at the campsite, dig a shallow pit in the ground and surround it with rocks. This fireproof border guards against the fire spreading out of control.

In rain or snow, begin a fire the same way. Twiggies, found on the lower trunks of trees, are almost always dry. The thick branches above absorb water and shelter them from moisture. However, plan on at least twice as many twiggies, pine needles, moss, or dead leaves as you would use during dry weather. Once a small fire of kindling is burning, firewood needs to be dried by the fire before fueling it. This is the reason for an increased amount of dry kindling. During heavy rain or snow, a fire needs constant attention and an endless supply of dry wood. It is best to wait until after the storm has passed before attempting to start a fire in a heavy downpour—a nearly impossible feat because each drop of water manages to put out that much flame.

Charcoal Lighter

Charcoal lighter fluid is a godsend for starting a warm, happy fire during a storm. Saturate an entire pile of medium-size branches with the lighter. Keeping a safe distance, throw a lighted match onto the wood. The flame will grow into a welcome fire almost immediately. The charcoal lighter soaks into the pores of the wood and holds the flame there long enough to ignite the wood. A small can of lighter fluid can be packed along under wet conditions. Where rain or snow is expected, some smart campers carry a supply of dry, split firewood. Once the basic fire is started with dry wood, the heat can quickly dry out wet wood, making it suitable for fuel.

Put a large log on the campfire before bedtime for a flicker of light and a comforting touch of warmth throughout the night. Then, in the morning, the fire can again be fed to its full strength without starting all over with kindling.

Upon leaving a campsite, pour water or dirt over the smoldering logs and separate the coals. Be certain the fire is out. Fire has an ugly way of spreading like a plague, despite the fact that you had to baby it to grow from a flame.

OUTDOOR EATING

The outdoors promotes an unhurried, lingering type of cooking and eating, in which preparation is as enjoyable as the eating. It is the joy of cooking and eating without worrying about the time and whether each course will be ready simultaneously. You eat because you are hungry but you cook as an exercise in woodswomanship, a living step in bringing you closer to nature.

Eating outdoors begins with planning at home. Plan each meal before leaving on vacation. Double-check that you have packed along the necessary ingredients. Stay with the plain and simple. The outdoors lends more to the food than any spice or sauce could ever hope to do. Food tastes better cooked outside the confines of four walls. Natural herbs and aromas seem to travel unseen through the air and enter the food, cooking it to perfection.

Even if you are not backpacking, include a dehydrated or freeze-dried meal. Quick and easy, such dishes nourish when the flesh is tired but the spirit cannot wait to move again. Think of tasty, spicy, one-dish dinners that the entire group relishes. Chili, stew, spaghetti, and macaroni and cheese with tuna save on pots as well as on the cook. Make them at home, freeze them and pack them in the cooler. They will defrost on the way and be ready when you are.

Campfire Cooking

Even though you should expect to do most of the cooking on the outdoor stove, plan to broil steaks, hamburgers, and chops over an open fire. This is easy without using a pan. Yet the smoky flavor makes the food special.

Grills. The trick of cooking over a campfire is really simple. Add a sizable portion of wood and wait for it to burn down to a bed of glowing red coals. Place a grill over the coals. The grill can be from an old refrigerator or stove, or an outdoor grill, available at sporting goods stores. Backpacking grills are about two feet long and six inches wide and fit into a backpack. Yet they provide a stable base for

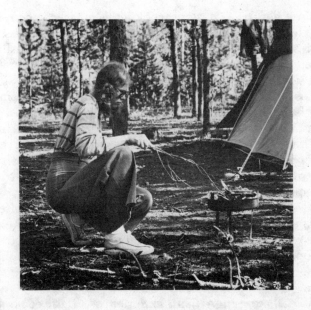

A modern substitute for glowing cooking coals in a campfire is charcoal briquets in a compact grill.

cooking over a campfire. Or you can build the fire between two large logs, a skillet size apart. Balance the pots and pans between the two logs over the cooking coals.

Charcoal Briquets.   A modern substitute for the glowing cooking coals is charcoal briquets. In a campsite with a grill but little firewood, charcoal briquets are the best way to build a cooking fire. Pile the briquets in pyramid fashion. Douse with charcoal lighter and ignite with a lighted match. When the coals become a red-gray color, spread the briquets flat for a larger cooking area, put on the grill and ready yourself for a thrilling cooking sensation.

When frying, boiling, or simmering over an open fire, place the skillet or pot over the coals and cook with careful attention. To prevent food from sticking, stir with a wooden spoon frequently. If the dish is cooking too fast, brush some of the coals to one side. If too slow, pile coals up higher underneath the pot.

Dutch Oven.   Outdoor cooking is nearly synonymous with dutch oven cookery. The dutch oven is a timeless, big, cast-iron pot with three small squat legs and a cover, slightly domed and with a lip standing up all along the outer edge. Even though a dutch oven weighs a little over sixteen pounds, it is worth the poundage and bulk when camping from horse panniers or a vehicle.

The dutch oven is famous for all-day stews. Put in the ingredients, dig a hole in the fire, and line it with coals. Lower the dutch oven into the hole, cover with coals and then dirt. Unearth it in four to six hours and eat a stew supreme with hardly any work.

The dutch oven lives up to its name when baking biscuits, cakes, and bread. Put in the dough; then surround the oven and cover the lid with coals. In this way, food is baked from the top, sides, and bottom. The even heat which cast iron promotes produces light and fluffy baked goods.

Basic Cooking Ingredients and Menus.   Basic cooking ingredients include Bisquick, liquid margarine, sugar, and seasonings (salt, pepper, chili powder, garlic and onion

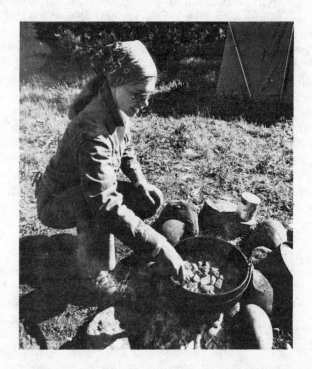

Outdoor cooking is nearly synonymous with dutch oven cookery.

powder, grated parmesan cheese, and honey in a squeeze tube). Use instant ingredients for cooking, such as instant milk and instant eggs, like Eggstra. Even though bacon and eggs can be savored for special days, instant cereal and dehydrated omelets with a freeze-dried bacon bar can be alternative breakfasts. Bisquick can be the basis of golden brown pancakes, plump, feathery-light biscuits, or the crisp coating for beer-batter deep-fried fresh fish fillets. Instant cocoa, tea, Tang, and fruit drinks can satisfy thirst as well as a craving for sweets.

Instant soup served with cheese, sausage, and crackers can make a delicious lunch. Top it off with gorp, a trail snack consisting of M&M candies, Spanish peanuts, raisins, and shredded coconut.

Supper will be consumed with gusto whether it be dehydrated lasagne with freeze-dried meatballs, grilled cheeseburgers, or homemade chili.

When planning each meal in the comfort of your kitchen, include a little extra food. Put all the rations that do not require refrigeration in one food bag, grub box, or container. This includes Bisquick, spices, eating utensils and plates, napkins, and instant ingredients. All boxed food (like macaroni and cheese dinner) should be removed from the container and packed in heavy-duty plastic bags for easy storing before you leave home. This procedure takes time but is practical for any camp cook who wants to be organized and not lose part of the supplies in a jumble in the trunk of the car. Backpackers repack foodstuffs into plastic bags out of necessity. It reduces weight as well as the amount of space items take up.

Store paper towels, pots, and skillet in a separate big box. The cooler contains perishables, like jelly, margarine, meat, pickles, catsup, and mustard. As items are used—for example, instant milk when preparing pancakes—close the plastic bag from which they are taken with a twist tie and replace them in the food bag. Taking time to put things back in their proper places will keep you organized and insures against insects invading or birds stealing them.

Build a fire slowly. Watch it grow and then dwindle into glowing coals. Mix pancakes in a pot and pour them sizzling onto a hot griddle. Smother them with liquid margarine and honey. Savor the tastes and aroma. Then, throw on some bacon and a few eggs. . . .

Fry battered fish fillets fresh from the lake. Eat them hot. Top the main course off with dehydrated hash-brown potatoes with your own touch of onion powder, grated parmesan cheese, and doses of pepper. . . .

Roast hot dogs over a fire on a green willow stick. Brown marshmallows on the same skewer. . . .

Anything your taste and imagination allow.

VENTURING AWAY FROM CAMP

Orienteering is a sport that involves finding your way through the wilderness by reading nature's signs. With map and compass, you decipher the way through unknown territory to an appointed destination. John Disley in his *Orienteering* (Stackpole, 1973) describes in detail the use of topographic maps and compass and how to practice these skills through orienteering.

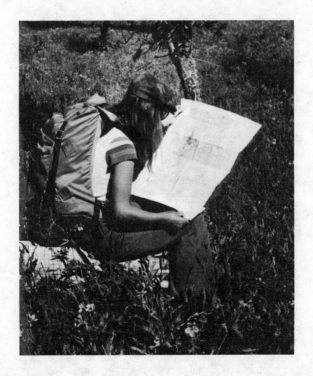

Acquaint yourself with reading topographic maps and compass. Orienteering is a sport that teaches you these skills.

Once you have mastered plotting your way on a map and following that route on an actual hike, the unmarked wilderness is yours to explore.

Outdoor skills help a woman achieve a level of self-sufficiency. They are something personal. Something of her own that she can recall at times when she needs reassurance of her own worth. She then will refuse to be lost in anyone's shadow. This is what involvement with the outdoors has given Joan Wulff and what is available to you too. "I have always worked on myself to get rid of hangups, to roll with the punch, to see the situation clearly and get on with the business of living without babying myself. I may not always succeed, but I'm trying." That is all anybody can ask and that is all nature wants. You, trying.

7

Personal Cleanliness and Grooming

Pregnant, life-sustaining, fertile. The earth. Upon her, living creatures, like you, walk, sleep, grow, reproduce. Generation after generation, she is stable, constant. Yet she is always changing, imperceptibly, and influencing those dependent on her to transform themselves into mature, fruitful organisms. Existence relies heavily on the earth. Yet she is taken for granted. She is overused and abused. Sometimes part of her dies from thirst or hunger. She is gouged, stripped, and dynamited. She suffers mistreatment, mismanagement, and misunderstanding. But the worst assault has been to call her rich soil "dirt."

The scourge of any housekeeper, dirt means unclean, filthy, stained. What three-year-olds have a genius for attracting. Dirt distinguishes the ignorant from the cultured, the haphazard from the meticulous, the careless from the thoughtful. Dirt often inflicts an aching feeling of guilt on housewives. The condition of being dirty was condemned by the Protestant ethic. Dirt on the exterior of a person meant that the soul, character, and temperament were probably likewise soiled. Dirty things could be expected from a dirty individual. And this, in turn, gave an immoral connotation to "dirt."

Even though soil and dirt are opposites, they are frequently confused. Clarification is needed. Dirt accompanies civilization; yet soil supports that civilization. Soil is clean and life-giving, whereas dirt is soot that smothers all that is shiny and white. Dirt is man-made but soil could have been created only by a higher Being. Dirt needs to be washed away, while soil requires tilling to bear fruit. Soil and dirt are divergent and should not even be mentioned in the same sentence. Yet people use the two terms interchangeably.

This mix-up is behind the mistaken impression that the outdoors is dirty. Mud, grass, weeds, sand, pebbles, and bugs are not dirt. And they do not make one dirty. They are natural participants in a living outdoors. As you are.

What is dirt to certain people, is a livelihood to others. Grease under the fingernails is disgraceful to the sanitary conscience of those who do not work with their hands. But to a mechanic, "dirty" fingernails mean a steady income and money in the bank. Clods of manure on a pair of boots are abhorrent to city dwellers. From the farmer's viewpoint, the smell of manure signifies home and prosperity. Ink-stained hands look disgusting to the uninitiated. However, they represent a hard day's work to the printer.

Dirt is subjective. One man's dirt is another's fortune. As Lee Marvin sang in the musical *Paint Your Wagon*, "The best things in life are dirty." Of course, he voiced this conviction because he associated gold with dirt and mud. When panning for gold, the dirt washes away, exposing nuggets of wealth. Dirt was not only tolerated, it was beloved for being the vehicle of discovery of gold.

Associating the outdoors with dirt can be a major factor in keeping a woman away from the backwoods. She imagines the outdoors crowded with creepy, crawly bugs that scamper across exposed flesh, causing a bad case of goosepimples. Or a film of sand covering the skin, producing a crunchy, grating sensation at the elbow, knee, ankle, and leg joints. Or mosquito bites the size of silver dollars inciting an uncontrollable urge to scratch. These can be

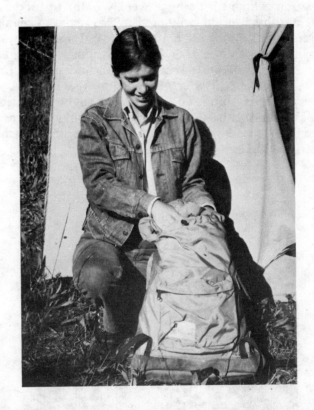

In the outdoors, the individual has power over the degree of comfort she enjoys.

prevented by using insect repellent, and by wearing slacks and long-sleeved shirts. But there is more to nature.

In the outdoors, just as at home, the individual has power over the degree of comfort she enjoys. But only by taking a chance and entering the backcountry can she realize how much control she has over the environment, even a wild one.

A REASONABLE STANDARD OF CLEANLINESS

Granted that the outdoors is not dirty, is it clean, you may ask. Can a beginner camper spend time in the backwoods without craving a bath? That depends on how fanatic the person is about a daily or weekly bath. In modern society, sterility is often promoted as "hygiene." Cleanliness is not enough. You must be spotless. And not merely your body but every dish, corner, cupboard, dog, lawn, and car around you. Smells and sweating are forbidden. Your breath should not be of onions or of medicine. It should be without a trace of anything. The entire body ought to be deodorized. Hair and teeth should be perfectly shiny and bright. By civilized standards, you and your environment should be sterile without a sanitary flaw.

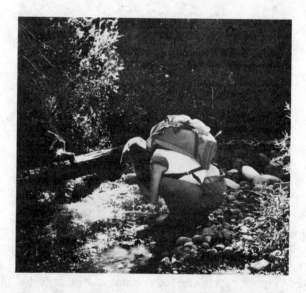

In the wilderness, water is a precious commodity and must be conserved. The camper should adopt a common-sense approach to personal hygiene.

It is impossible to maintain these standards in the wilds. Without running water, a sink, shower, and bathtub, it is impractical. The backpacker hauls water from a nearby stream in a one-gallon plastic bag. Considerable effort is involved in accumulating enough water to prepare dinner and wash the eating and cooking utensils. A tubful of water is out of the question. The backpacker needs to conserve both water and fuel. With a very limited supply, drinking water and food preparation come first. Spotlessness does not even enter the mind.

Even at an organized campground where the precious liquid comes from a faucet, the water must be carried to the campsite. This limits the available supply and imposes natural restrictions on the amount of water that can be used. However, if the campground has restroom and shower facilities, home cleansing rituals can be carried over to the camping situation without problems. The farther away from civilization, the more practical one must be about sanitary conditions.

Before entering the wilderness, the outdoorswoman should realize she cannot practice the grooming ceremony she is accustomed to at home. By adopting a common-sense approach to personal hygiene, however, she can feel reasonably clean and comfortable in the bush.

BATHS AND SHOWERS

In the backcountry, a daily bath or shower is out of the question. Going a week or two without a bath is common and part of the total experience. It is a complete departure from civilization, and bathlessness helps make the trip unusual and memorable. It is fun to rebel against the unwritten sanitary laws of society.

Most soaps pollute streams, ponds, and lakes (Ivory soap is one of the best "natural" soaps). In addition, "biodegradable" soaps are relatively new on the market. Although they claim they do not pollute the environment, do not trust them. Rinse water is unnatural to the waterway's balance. It contaminates.

Sponge Baths

Into the backwoods, pack along a plastic basin. The size depends on the amount of room available in the backpack. From the bowl, you can scoop water up with both hands and splash your face. Be sure it is large enough. It will serve as a bathtub and double as a portable dishwashing sink. From it, an exhilarating sponge bath is possible.

Fill the basin with water. Find a secluded, sunny spot behind a boulder or a cluster of Engelmann spruce. Take off your clothes and hang them over the boulder or branches of trees to air out.

A sponge bath is more exciting to take than a quick dip in a lake. Here you are exposed. Peering stealthily from your hiding place, you feel daring and a touch evil. Wearing not a stitch, you are as free as wildlife. You wish a deer would appear next to you. Would it notice that you are naked? The sun is so warm, you want to lie against the heated rock. Each pore soaks up ultraviolet light, transmitting energy.

An urge to run strikes. You bolt from the hideaway. But the pebble- and sagebrush-studded ground prohibits barefoot travel. Unshackled in the open air. No doors, no locks, no walls, no mirrors. With arms outspread, stretch to touch the sky, extend to the four corners of the world. The earth is your mother. You stand unafraid without hiding, completely vulnerable.

A brisk breeze rustles the distant aspens. Once again you jump behind the large rock for protection. The wind encircles your body, leaving goosebumps all over. Each inch of skin shivers under the stirring air. Seductive. No part is covered up. Everything, revealed. No shame. Completely receptive. This must be how Eve felt.

With only one pan of water, use soap sparingly. Otherwise, a film of soap will be left on the skin. Some ambitious bathers fill the basin and one or two cooking pots with water. When the basin's water turns a milky white, they throw it on the ground, at least twenty feet from the stream. Fresh water reinforcements from the pots are then poured into the bowl. It takes more planning and effort but ensures a thorough rinsing.

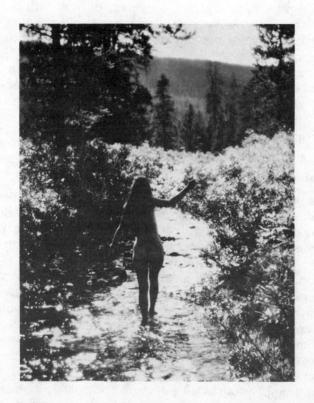

Wearing not a stitch, you are as free as wildlife.

A sponge bath is not as relaxing as a tub bath. On the contrary, it rouses. But one is as effective as the other. You wash away bacteria and the stickiness left behind by strenuous exercise and perspiration. A sponge bath is primarily a physical sensation. The senses are not dulled by a pool of water. The slightest change in the atmosphere produces a wave of feeling from the eyebrows through the torso down to the toenails.

Frontier Indians believed that dunking themselves daily in a nearby stream caused their blood to run faster and made them stronger, more alert with quicker reflexes. Braves performed this ritual in the winter as well as the summer. They chopped a hole in the ice and jumped into the frigid water. Squaws, however, did not bathe as frequently. They were considered cowards by being born female and were not subjected to physical trials as proof of courage.

The equipment necessary for a sponge bath is a basin with water, a washcloth or sponge, a bar of soap—one without phosphates—and a towel. A hand towel takes up less space and does the job of drying; a bath-size towel is a luxury.

Natural and Improvised Showers

Rain is the natural shower. Unfortunately, cool temperatures and a chilly breeze often accompany rain. But on those occasions when a light drizzle and warm air combine for the perfect conditions, take advantage of the situation and shower. Scamper through a grassy meadow, picking wild flowers while the sprinkle of water droplets dots your skin with moisture and washes away the residue of exertion. Dripping from your eyebrows into the eyes, the rivulets of water make your pores feel alive and moving. It is the ultimate of exhilaration.

If you are not lucky enough to capture nature at the right moment, create your own shower. Carry along a three-pound empty coffee can punctured with ice pick holes on the bottom. Near the top on opposite sides of the can, punch two more holes. Through these insert a section of nylon ropes used as a handle. Wrap the handle around the branch of a tree and hang the container high enough to stand under. Ideally, a friend pours water into the can while you scrub vigorously under the dribbling shower. It is possible, however, if you are alone, to pour the water and scrub simultaneously. It is not nearly as pleasurable as a shower shared with a companion.

Depending on the dedication of the friend, the shower is usually short but invigorating. Devoted friends have been known to heat the water before pouring, but these are hard to find. When your shower is over, it is the friend's turn and you are the laborer. Mutual shower-giving helps build an intimate working relationship.

Outdoor showers can highlight a trip. While they are fun and stimulating, they also are a luxury and can involve hard work hauling water. They are not absolutely necessary for a week's trek but they bring companions close.

Wintertime Bathing

While camping in cold temperatures, avoid wetting any part of the body. Cold water chills the entire body even if it is applied only to the face and hands. In freezing temperatures, it can lead to frostbite. Most winter campers insulate the body against the cold by wearing a layer of long underwear at all times. To them, warmth is more vital than washing.

However, washing the face can be refreshing and lift the spirit during a particularly bleak blizzard. And cooks should wash their hands before preparing meals. There is a way to cleanse hands, face, and any other part of the body without soap, water, and towel. Use Wet Ones. These are small towelettes, presaturated with a cleansing lotion. They clean the skin, leaving a fresh aroma behind. The skin dries quickly without chapping. Other types of cleansing tissues are on the market, but these are the only ones with a handy pop-up dispenser.

With Wet Ones, water does not need to be hauled. Fuel is not expended to heat up the water. Soap, washcloth, and towel are eliminated. Wet Ones are convenient face and hand cleaners during summer camping too. The used towelette is thrown into the fire and disintegrates. Washing is quick and easy. Not as soothing as a bath or shower, the towelettes are trouble-free cleansers when time or weather makes bathing impractical.

CARE OF THE TEETH

Bring along a toothbrush and small tube of toothpaste. Brushing your teeth in the morning chases away "dragon mouth" and reassures you that you are taking care of yourself. Cleaning the teeth at night helps to prepare you for bed. Sleep seems to come easier. Half a teaspoon of salt in a glass of water is an effective mouthwash. These are also the times when moist towelettes can cleanse the face and hands. Pampering yourself in these ways is a touch of civilization that produces a sense of well-being by reminding you that out beyond this wilderness lies familiar society.

MAKEUP

Forget the mirror. Without a mirror, you worry less about your appearance. As a result, you primp less and are more concerned with your surroundings than with yourself. "Take me as I am," you tell the world and whomever you meet along the way. In a mirrorless culture, you realize how much time, energy, and money are wasted on appearance.

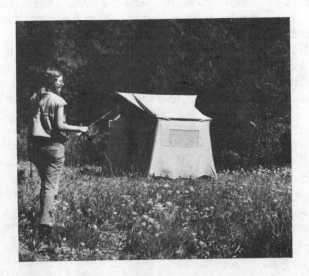

Forget mirror and makeup. You then are more concerned with your surroundings than with yourself.

Mascara, powder, eyeliner, eyebrow pencil, lipstick, blush-on are all omitted. More time is left to soak in the good things around you. As you become less self-conscious, others seem to relax and feel at home with you. What a realization: You are you—attractive even without makeup.

Are you appalled by the idea of forgetting the makeup kit? Then bring it along. See how troublesome and out of place it is. Chances are you will leave it at home on the next trip.

HAIR

A hair-do will flop in the outdoors. Be aware of this fact ahead of time. No amount of coddling will salvage it. Nature is used to fur, feathers, and scales. Ducks and geese preen and humans comb. That is the extent of the assistance an outdoorswoman can lend to disarrayed hair.

The extremes of short or long hair are easiest to take care of. Short hair looks natural and attractive wind-blown. A once-through with a brush revives it. Long hair, on the other hand, can be pulled back by a rubber band or tied into braids or pony tails. Tangles do not occur because the hair is tight against the head, out of reach of the wind.

Medium-length hair is the most bothersome. Too long to let it wave in the wind. Too short to control with a rubber band. A scarf or hat is the only answer. A bandana tied peasant-style at the base of the neck tames the hair and shelters it from sun and dust. Cotton does not slip off the head as readily as nylon or other synthetic material. A bright-colored neckerchief enlivens the face, bringing a blush to the cheeks and dazzle to the eyes.

Do not expect to wash your hair in the backwoods. Hair washing requires too much water for adequate rinsing. It involves extra work and wastes a limited water supply. The threat of chill while the hair is drying is always present and can cause a severe cold. Covering the hair with scarf or hat keeps the hair cleaner longer. An outdoorswoman can go without a shampoo for as long as two weeks. Even though she would like to wash her hair, it is not a major problem that she cannot.

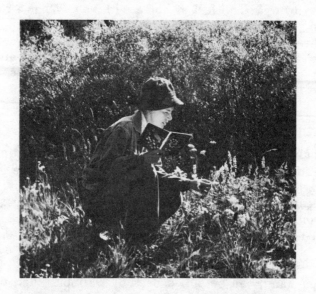

To protect the hair from sun and dirt, wear a hat.

BODY CARE

Using a deodorant daily in the backwoods is a must. Physically more active, the body perspires more on a camping trip. Even in cold weather, clothes trap perspiration next to the skin. Without a deodorant, body odor can be a problem. You wish you could climb out of yourself.

Q-tips or swabs are plastic toothpicks with cotton at each end. They are handy at home to clean children's nose and ears. They are also useful for the outdoorswoman to remove wax from ears, which builds up to a greater extent in the outdoors.

Face, arms, and hands, exposed to the sun most of the day on the trail, can become tenderly dry. Suntan lotion or a medicated moisture cream can bring instant, welcomed relief. Chapstick soothes chapped, parched lips in a similar manner.

Feet and Nails

To a hiker, feet are vital. More valuable than camping gear, topographic maps, compass, and food. Feet should be in prime condition for extended treks—dry, blister- and corn-free, and groomed. A backpacker should pamper the feet.

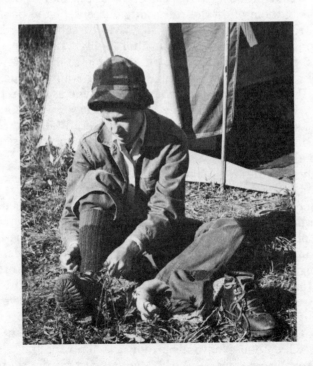

Feet are essential to a hiker. Pamper them.

Initially, invest in a pair of quality hiking boots (see Chapter 3) made of leather with Vibram soles and ankle and foot support. While wearing two pairs of wool socks, choose the boots to fit comfortably, not too snug. Do not wear cotton or nylon socks even in the summer. On a hot, dusty trail, the feet sweat. Wool absorbs perspiration yet ventilates the feet. Cotton and nylon become saturated with perspiration, preventing the feet from drying off. Wearing wet cotton or nylon socks is like walking in water. The feet lose color from inadequate circulation and wrinkle from overexposure to moisture. Within three days, a fungus invades the feet.

When the feet are damp, wash and dry them as soon as possible. Wet socks and shoes irritate the feet, facilitating the formation of blisters. At the nearest source of water, relax. Take off boots and socks. Wiggle the toes in the grass and cool them off in the refreshing current. If the boots are wet from wading, particles of gravel or sand settle inside them at the bottom. Wash thoroughly. Likewise, rinse socks. Dry feet with scarf or handkerchief. Change to clean wool socks. Fresh socks are soothing therapy to tuckered feet. If dry clean socks are not available, you are ill-prepared and will be less comfortable. In such a case, wring out the wet socks and put them back on dry feet. Walking will be like sloshing around in a bog but the feet will be less damaged than with soggy socks. Treat your feet lovingly and gently and they will serve you faithfully and well.

For hot, aching feet, remove boots and socks and fan the tender skin cool. Massage your arches. When feet become hot and tired, the fun evaporates from a hike. The condition of the feet directly influences the attitude of the backpacker. Gauge your pace according to what your feet are telling you. Feet do not lie. After a rest, reverse the socks: put the right one on the left foot and vice versa. This procedure stimulates the feet and guards against holes wearing through the socks.

Cut toenails short. Long, jagged toenails can cut into toes, which can eventually produce a limp for the camper without a nail clipper. A tiny toenail can be the source of pain that infects the entire body.

Fingernail polish is out of place in the backcountry. Manicures are impractical but groomed nails can be accomplished with an emory board or nail file. Anything beyond that is uncalled for.

FIRST AID

Even though the chances of injury are slight, the camper should be prepared. Cuts to hands and fingers are the most frequent type of physical mishap in the outdoors. These result from a haphazard use of knives and axes. Caution can prevent them. For cuts, bring a small shatterproof bottle or tube of antiseptic, such as hydrogen peroxide or first aid cream.

When trudging through heavy brush, twigs from nearby bushes and trees can scrape the unprotected eye. In addition, seeds from weeds fly about madly when disturbed. One of these can lodge in the eye. While these are not serious injuries, they can cause irritation and hamper vision. For these, a medicated eye ointment can reduce inflammation and wash the foreign particle from the eye.

The backwoods is inhabited by more insects than any other type of wildlife. And they are usually most active during the summer, when most people have an opportunity to enter the wilds. An insect repellent helps prevent stings and bites. Each area of the country seems to have its own favorite type of repellent. The Rockies, for instance, favor Cutter's lotion while the Southwest seems to endorse Off insect spray.

Occasionally, campers suffer stings and bites despite efforts to protect themselves. A paste of baking soda and water—a family remedy for at least a century—reduces swelling and irritation. Outdoor lore traditionally prescribes mud for insect bites. The last resort is soaking in water. Terrestrial insects drown when they hit water. If the swarms are too bad, dunk yourself in the nearest pool and stay until dark. Generally, pesky insects are not as active in the cool of night.

Baking soda (1/4 teaspoon in 1/2 glass of water) also soothes indigestion.

With the amount of exercise a camper engages in outdoors, irregularity of bowels is usually a far-fetched notion. However, if this happens to be the case, a rounded teaspoon of salt in a quart of warm water taken on an empty stomach will do wonders. Lomotil tablets, prescribed by a physician prior to the trip, are an effective remedy for diarrhea.

Band-aids, adhesive tape, and gauze bandages are essential in binding blisters against further irritation. They cover cuts and minor wounds and guard against infiltration by insects and soil particles.

A pair of tweezers is necessary to remove a splinter without using a knife. More than likely, at least one splinter will annoy you each trip.

Pack the soap, lotion, Chapstick, medicated cream, and other items in one small nylon pouch. Everything will be in easy reach, organized in one location. Nothing lost.

Feminine hygiene is simple outdoors. Easier than it ever is in society. In the woods, reasonably clean is the rule. In civilization, a woman strives for beauty, using the latest Rubenstein eyeshadow, lip and rouge color. But a human cannot equal the spectacular panorama of nature, no matter how much makeup is applied. That is reassuring, comforting to a woman. She needs to be only herself.

Natural, that is the key.

8

Feminine Hygiene

Skin against skin. Two bodies intertwined. Layers of wool, the thick loft of goose down, electric blankets, battery-operated foot warmers, catalytic heaters—nothing can surpass the warmth generated from two humans loving.

With your own Robert Redford, you are thrilled, comforted, wanted, needed. Stroking his sandy hairs, looking behind the ocean-blue eyes, you float attached into the untainted atmosphere. Together you soar above the shimmering lake, alive with feeding brook trout, and see the aqua backpack tent below. The flexible walls of bliss, of unearthly pleasure, pushing all else from the mind. Propelled as a spirit, soaking in the nectar of the natural world, by the magic meeting of two earth-bound creatures. Flying high on the wings of screaming sensation. Taking off beyond human into the realm of transcending consciousness. The meeting of souls.

You are producing your own nature film. Funny how you are doing and watching at the same time. Clinging to each other, touching the very lifeline, it is both of you as one against the world. This way, nothing is more important than union. Troubles are insignificant. Bring on any challenge. Nobody, no happening can penetrate the bond.

Nature is the best place to do what comes naturally. A headache, tired muscles, sore feet are soothed, caressed away by making love in the outdoors. At an isolated spot, the stars make a spectacular canopy. Drown petty irritations in an explosion of physical sensation. Put things where they belong. Expose yourself to the wilds. It was meant to be that way.

Historically, women have thrived in the so-called hard life of the outdoors. Sacajawea, a Shoshone Indian, is probably one of the most familiar female names in early western history. She was sixteen years old and pregnant when her husband, Charbonneau, a French trader, signed a contract attaching them to the Lewis and Clark expedition as interpreters. While preparing for the long journey, Sacajawea

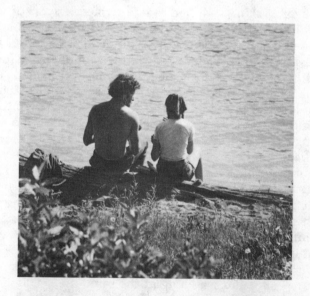

Nature is the best place to do what comes naturally.

suffered a prolonged labor. Fearing for the squaw's life, a trader tried an old Indian remedy—the rattles from a rattlesnake crumbled into a glass of water. Ten minutes after drinking the mixture, Sacajawea gave birth to a son.

For seventeen months, she, her husband, and son Baptiste accompanied Lewis and Clark on their pathfinding explorations of 1805 and 1806. During this time, nursing was the only source of nourishment for the baby. Sacajawea carried the infant in a woven basket on her back. She wrapped him in moss which was highly absorbent and served as diapers. Exposed to near-starvation, cold, wet weather, and back-breaking hauling of canoes and gear, both mother and child remained healthy. Illness struck Sacajawea twice; the baby only once. In contrast, the men endured much physical pain—boils, influenza, and dysentery.

On the trail, life goes on. Babies are conceived. Love is enkindled. Emotions boil. Hikers grow up. Wisdom blooms. The outdoors is an integral part of it all, even if your world revolves around the city. Nature is central to existence. To separate what ties you to the earth from what attracts you to neon lights is like trying to separate scent from flowers. When one part of an organism is underdeveloped, the whole suffers.

Existence in the wilds can be painful and full of trials. But over the years, women have proven they can meet the challenge. On July 12, 1864, nineteen-year-old Mrs. Fanny Kelly was captured west of Fort Laramie by a band of Ogalalla Sioux. She was traveling to Idaho with an emigrant train from her home in Kansas. The Indians released her at Fort Sully in the Dakota Territory five months later.

In her book, *My Captivity Among the Sioux* (Corinth Books, 1962), she described her fears, periodic mistreatment, and customs of the Indians. At first, the Sioux forced her into submission by strictly rationing food and water intake. Gradually, the Indian women accepted her as the chief's fourth wife. As squaws are expected to do, she performed heavy manual chores. In short, she adapted remarkably well during only five months of tepee living, even to the extent of learning the Indian tongue.

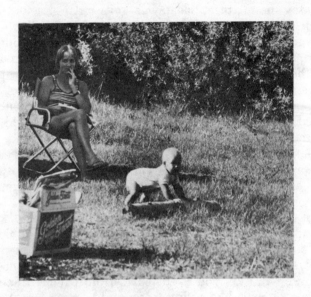

On the trail, life goes on.

The Indians brought her to Fort Sully as a decoy. The band hoped to get inside the fort and slaughter the soldiers. The plan was squelched. The fort gate closed behind the white woman and the chief, blockading the braves.

At this time in history, pioneers were carving a livelihood out of the frontier. To them, wilderness, weather, and wildlife were to be conquered. They viewed a rocky section of sagebrush as a challenge. Either they cleared it and raised crops and livestock, or they lost, possibly died. They fought the wilds daily. The main goal was to build a town worth putting on the map—another Saint Louis or Sante Fe. So deeply entrenched in nature, they were striving for civilization. Without conveniences and with a rifle as their only protection, they yearned for the day when they could rest, experience comfort, and enjoy what they worked so hard to get.

While romanticists in the city pictured the Indian as a "noble savage," the frontierspeople saw him as a killer, a pillager, a destroyer. The Indian personified the wilderness —strange, unknown, and unpredictable. Within a "proper society" was where white man belonged. Pioneers joined forces for protection against massacre by the Indians.

Against this background and imbued with intense hatred of the red man, Fanny Kelly found herself alone, at the mercy of people she assumed were devilish and sadistic. During the three hundred years of American frontier life, innumerable women were captured by Indians. Some perished but most of them married braves and reared children. A few like Fanny Kelly were fortunate enough to return to white civilization. All of them felt a degree of kinship for the tribal, primitive existence.

Only within the past hundred years have Americans decided that their rightful place is inside four walls. Before that, Americans sought new frontiers to settle. Because towns have crowded out most unexplored land, many persons fail to see the value of nature. To be, to do, to care— these are treasures the outdoors offers the outdoorsperson. To be yourself. To do what is natural. To care for the wild things. This is how women in the past survived the rigors of nature. Today, this is the only way to maintain nature for tomorrow.

Make love in the outdoors. Dedicate it to the perpetual procreation of nature.

MENSTRUATION

The body's processes go on, even though you are out of the familiar, convenient environment of home, hiking a chunk of national forest. When it is time, menstruation will occur whether you are prepared for it or not, no matter where you are.

When feminine hygiene is discussed, a woman generally thinks first of the menstrual period. The way she speaks of this monthly biological phenomenon reflects how she expects to be treated by others and what levels of cleanliness she demands during these five to seven days. Whether the menstrual period is called "a curse," "my friend," or "my period" is important in determining the level of adjustment the woman can make outdoors at this time of the month.

A woman who thinks the menstrual period is a curse will have difficulty in behaving in a normal way during menstruation. She sees herself as inferior to men, and believes that she is being punished for an unknown transgression. She is usually ignorant of the biological facts behind menstruation and engages in a type of fantasy that Sigmund Freud described as "penis envy." She is a critical, rigid individual who believes she must go through one week of hell each month. This woman is in the minority, fortunately, and would most likely seldom be inclined to venture into the wilderness. If she did, she should be a member of a class or group with knowledgeable leaders and plan the trip carefully so as to avoid being afield during menses.

"My friend" is an ironical name for menstruation. On the one hand, menstruation identifies the female as mature and fertile. It is predictable—probably one of the few things that is—and hardly ever lets her down. On the other hand, menses slows down the woman. In her mind, she is not herself during this time. She is inhibited by a natural process which men do not have to suffer. She feels unclean and weak. In a sense, she feels she is biologically vulnerable during this week because of loss of lifeblood. For this reason, she takes medication and pampers herself as if she were sick. This exaggeration is more common among women than the curse theme is.

The female camper with "my friend" along will find the outdoors trying and exhausting. She needs to engage in an activity, like fishing or swimming, that will preoccupy her thoughts without allowing the dread of menstruation to enter. Cramps can be worked out through walking and staying active. Remaining in the tent all day merely intensifies them. At bedtime, one or two aspirins or menstrual medication can be taken. But during the day, these types of pills can produce sluggishness, especially when the backpacker is engaged in strenuous exercise.

Calling menstruation "my period" is merely an abbreviation of "my menstrual period" and most women classify it in this manner. That is, a cyclic biological process, like digestion, natural as the wilderness itself. This woman will have little if any adjustment to make outdoors during menstruation.

Feminine hygiene during menstruation becomes more of a problem the longer the backcountry trip. On day-long hikes without an overnight stop, the camper can bring a change of protection—either a sanitary napkin or a tampon. On extended backpack trips, however, the space and weight factors become critical. Then, a decision should be made about the most desirable type of protection.

Sanitary Napkins vs. Tampons

Sanitary napkins are big, bulky, and hard to dispose of. Tampons are more convenient, easier to store, take up less space, and are simpler to dispose of. They are also more comfortable when walking long distances. On a seven-day backpack trip the camper expecting her menstrual period should plan on packing and using about four tampons per day. While old wives' tales warn that exercise increases the amount of menstrual flow, science disagrees. The number of tampons used each day in the wilderness will be approximately the same as that needed while at home.

Tampons are useful to absorb a flow other than menstruation. After making love, before climbing into the sleeping bag, insert a tampon. This eliminates the clammy wetness that would otherwise permeate the sleeping bag for the rest of the night, producing a restless sleep.

The Menstrual Cup

A third alternative is the menstrual cup. Women in the Peace Corps, stationed in the Far East, report the cup is convenient and economical. Simply rinse in water and put it back in position. Like a diaphragm, use the cup repeatedly, thus eliminating the need for an extra supply. Also available is a type of menstrual cup that is effective for only about twelve hours, which makes it more expensive and less practical than other modes of protection.

Disposal of tampons or pads is the biggest problem in menstrual sanitation. The best way is by burning. Several studies into bear behavior have shown that the bruins are apparently attracted by them. Thus, complete incineration is necessary for safety in bear country as well as cleanliness.

Substitute for Douching

Douching is central to feminine hygiene. However, without a source of running water, a douche is impractical. Instead, sit in the middle of a stream. The current acts as a whirlpool, cleansing as well as soothing. The action of the water serves as a natural douche. Paraphernalia, such as hot water bags, are not needed.

During menstruation, bathing may be of paramount importance to a woman (see Chapter 7). But in the backcountry, a bath or shower may be equally impractical. The temperature may dip to forty each night and mosquitoes or black flies may attack any uncovered part of the body. The packer should consider this before leaving the trailhead. If a soothing bath is absolutely necessary for peace of mind and feeling at the peak of physical stamina, then the trek should be postponed. Before such a decision is reached, however, which in reality bans you from the pleasures of the wilds one week out of every four, consider the type of protection you use.

Sanitary napkins seem to make women feel dirtier than tampons do. The reason? Possibly because the pad is external to the body. The flow than is in contact with the outside of the body and when the discharge meets air, an odor is produced.

In contrast, a tampon is internal. It touches neither the skin nor the air. It eliminates the odor and the physical sensation of pad touching skin which is a constant reminder that menses are in progress. In fact, some women forget completely about menstruation after inserting a tampon. How is this possible? The old saying, "Out of sight, out of mind," may be partly responsible. Whatever the reason, cases have been reported of women complaining of a "vaginal growth." On further investigation, doctors have found forgotten tampons.

A number of women have an irrational fear of tampons, largely stemming from their mothers' attitude based on ignorance. Tampons are easy to insert and cannot be "lost" inside you. Because of the way the human female body is constructed, the tampon is "trapped" within the vagina. It cannot enter the tiny opening of the uterus. So, if the tampon should somehow push deeper into the vagina, bringing the dislodging string with it, you can reach up into the vagina, find the tampon and pull it out with your fingers. This happens infrequently.

Many outdoorswomen participate on two-week wilderness camping trips during menstruation and do not shower the entire time. With spirits high and energy pulsating, they look forward to a steaming hot bath when they return home.

Improvised Protection

What happens if your period occurs unexpectedly and you did not bring along any form of protection? Then use what is available, as the pioneer and Indian women did. Fold a piece of cloth—an extra pair of panties, a sock, a handkerchief—and place inside the undies, serving as a type of primitive sanitary napkin. If you have two safety pins, secure the pad to the underpants to prevent slippage.

Until the 1930s, this method was used by women. They folded a piece of sheet and pinned it to the panties. The fragment of material was not disposable. After being used once, it was soaked in bleach and sudsy water, laundered, and then reused. Admittedly, by modern standards, this type of menstrual protection can be considered crude. Feminine hygiene was nearly ignored by manufacturers until the 1920s. Then the taboo of mentioning such personal things in public was relaxed somewhat. Truly, women have come a long way in achieving proper consideration and recognition. But, in terms of the outdoors, a long, steep trail challenges woman. Determination will take her to the summit and her rightful place. It is waiting for you.

Long ago, Indian mothers discovered that moss serves as a convenient, efficient natural diaper. In a similar way, they probably took advantage of the absorbent qualities of moss for their own personal needs.

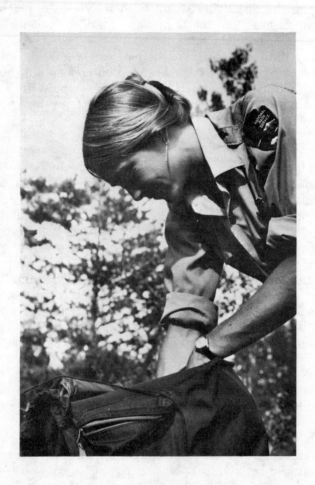

Wilderness travel makes you improvise. If you are not adequately prepared, use what you have in your backpack. Make do with available
provisions.

The most attractive aspect of wilderness travel is what it does to you. It makes you improvise. The menstrual period which has happened nearly every month since your thirteenth birthday suddenly takes on new dimensions. When away from the comforts of society, what should you do to keep yourself feeling clean and healthy? The menstrual period can be a problem while you are in the backwoods or it can be another challenge, forcing you into doing the same old thing in an entirely different way. All of a sudden, menstruation *means* something. Menses or not, you find you are clean of mind and spirit. Really clean!

THE OPEN AIR BATHROOM

Many newcomers to the outdoors are appalled by the lack of indoor plumbing, specifically, bathroom and toilet. But when you learn the "behind the bush" routine and overcome the initial shyness, you will actually prefer the open air bathroom to the outhouses found at "primitive campgrounds."

Using nature's toilet facilities is simple and invigorating. Find a protective bush and dig a small hole with the heel of the hiking boot. For compacted, hard soil, a sturdy folding shovel is better. A cavity approximately six inches deep is big enough. Chemicals in the topsoil break down the waste and use it as fertilizer. A hole deeper than six inches bypasses the topsoil. Beneath the top layer of earth, the disintegrating chemicals are not as abundant. The waste would not be dissolved or be transformed into fertilizer as quickly.

The squat position is difficult for many campers. It puts strain on the leg muscles and can be quite uncomfortable. When the muscles are quivering from exertion, the entire experience can be dreadful. Experienced outdoorswomen locate a bush or tree that provides support as well as privacy. Balance by holding onto a low branch and situate yourself over the depository. Or, like expert, skillful backwoodswomen, find a deadfall log which supports hips and upper legs while the buttocks extend over the log above the

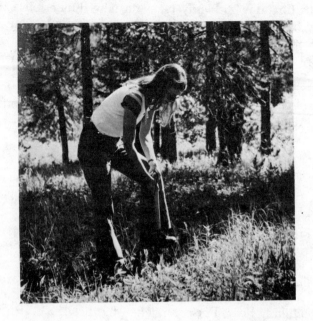

The open air bathroom sometimes requires a little digging.

freshly dug toilet. In terms of woodswomanship, this is the ultimate in planning and comfort when it is needed the most.

Toilet paper is too flimsy for outdoor usage. Facial tissues are more sturdy and are biodegradable. Deposit used tissues in the hole, unless a fire is handy. Then, burn the paper. Here also a tampon or sanitary napkin can be deposited; the cavity may have to be bigger for a sanitary napkin.

Cover the hole with soil and stomp the loose dirt down. The open bathroom can be anywhere. Exercise discretion. Choose a spot far enough from the campsite where no one is likely to redig the same hole. Be sure it is at least twenty feet away from a water source, to avoid contamination of creeks and lakes.

Feminine hygiene involves a relationship between woman and nature. On the one hand, a camper can find solace in the outdoors while undergoing menstruation and other biological functions. However, the woodswoman has a responsibility to leave no trace of her presence behind. Burn tissues, pads, and other waste items where possible. If burning is out of the question, burying is the second best method. Elk, deer, and moose pellets; raccoon scats, and coyote droppings are all part of the natural scheme. Human excrement and garbage are disgraces. While humans are creatures of nature, they have a duty to use common sense and care when dealing with the natural environment.

A woman can find a whole new panorama of sensations outside four walls. Nature is the right backdrop for what comes naturally. You are there, awed over the difference the outdoors makes in you.

9

Keeping a Clean Camp

The sun is so bright, the eyes squint behind dark glasses. Summer is young. Islands of encrusted snow dot the landscape as reminders of a harsher time when nature tested her creatures. Plants are just coming alive, pushing back the dull, buckskin layer of dead vegetation. Luminous yellow-green shoots promise colorful, heated days ahead.

This is the first backpack trip of the year. The trail is soggy in spots. Mud clings to the Vibram soles. Traction is annihilated. Trying to hike, you skate over the wet ground. The trek is easy, planned to reintroduce leg and back muscles to the rigors of the outdoors a little at a time.

Coming across a community of naked aspens and cottonwoods, just beginning to bud, your mind registers, "This would be a great campsite." Common sense double-checks first impressions, "Is there any water here? Camping without water is like buying an ice cream cone without ice cream."

On minitrips into popular park areas, water spigots are provided. Generally, a sign indicates whether the water is "safe drinking water" or "unsafe for drinking." Contaminated water is fine for bathing but it is unsatisfactory—even dangerous—for brushing teeth, dishwashing, and preparing food.

WATER CONTAINERS

A heavy, plastic, collapsible one-gallon water bag is handy for hauling drinking water from the source to the campsite. When empty, it compresses into a very small size—perfect for backpacking. To quench thirst on the trail, pack one or two pint-size, wide-mouthed plastic bottles with screw tops full of water. Refill them whenever possible. There are a lot of hiking trails, even in the mountains, that are devoid of good drinking water. To prevent dehydration, you must pack your own water.

For a camper who travels by car or horse, clean, plastic

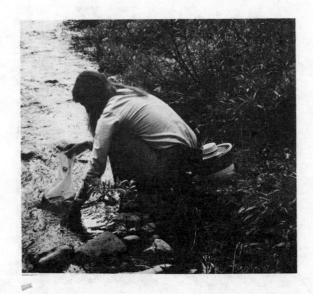

A heavy plastic collapsible water bag is handy for hauling water.

jerry cans or commercially manufactured water jugs take a lot of work out of hauling water. Practical water containers range from two to five gallons and eliminate repeated visits to the water source.

WATER SOURCES IN THE MOUNTAINS

From a water standpoint, most mountain areas are ideal for wilderness backpacking. Rivers begin in the mountains. Melting snow and rainwater trickle down steep crevices to form brooks. Eventually various brooks unite and grow into significant streams and rivers. Moisture likewise permeates porous rock and soil, creating underground springs. Gravity directs the flow of water downward to the valleys

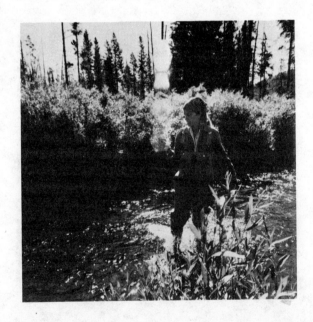

The headwaters of a river can be found in the mountains.

and plains. As creeks join at lower elevations, water volume increases, producing a strong current and powerful flood of life-giving, sustaining water.

The headwater or beginning of any river consists of a rivulet of water. The Snake River, for example, begins in Yellowstone National Park. There, it looks insignificant. Too shallow to contain large fish. Too narrow to amount to anything. Before the Snake slithers out of Yellowstone, however, it has been transformed into a mighty torrent. In fact, immediately out of Yellowstone, the Snake rages through Flagg Canyon, a narrow gorge where waves jump eight feet during high water in early summer. Floaters thrill at the risks involved in trying to master this part of the Snake—even if it is just a newborn babe.

Headwaters are pure, directly from mother nature. The closer the backpacker camps to the headwaters, the more chaste the water. Sucking up water directly from the stream is like nursing at nature's breast. The more a section is frequented by livestock and humans, the better the chance of pollution. If a horsepack group is headquartered upstream from you, do not trust the water, even though you are high in the mountains. However, if they are situated downstream, drink without fear. (Upstream is the direction from which the stream is coming. Downstream is where the stream is going.)

In unfamiliar country, a topographic or aerial map pinpoints water sources. Then, it is a matter of plotting the course from your location to the water by compass or landmarks. Since gravity draws water towards lower elevations, canyons and valleys are likely places to find water. From the vantage of a mountain peak, the careful eye can spot slivers of water sparkling in the sun.

An abundance of healthy trees, green bushes, blooming wild flowers, and lush plant life signifies the presence of water. It might not be on the surface. Dig a small hole in soft, moist ground and watch the cavity fill with water. Wait for the soil to settle to the bottom and drink freely. Even if a few soil particles are suspended in the water, it is safe. Nothing can be finer than water directly from earth's natural well.

WATER SOURCES IN THE DESERT

Availability of water should be a prime consideration when planning any camping trip, but it is especially critical when exploring the desert. In arid terrain, water is essential. Without it, energy is sapped quickly. The tongue feels swollen several sizes too large for the mouth. Cool, refreshing water obsesses the mind. In short, without water in the desert, a carefree excursion turns into an ugly survival test.

Before entering desert country, be sure of the water supply. In a vehicle, where weight is not a deterrent, load enough water to allow for three gallons of water per person per day. This is the minimum daily requirement without sacrificing. On foot, carry one gallon per person for each day. While this amount does not demand rationing, it requires conservative use. Consider that a gallon of water weighs 8⅓ pounds. Multiply this by the number of days you plan to explore the desert. The result is the total weight of an adequate water supply. You will likely cut your trip in half. Packing water on your back, in addition to other supplies, produces an enormous poundage. This more than any other factor limits the popularity of desert backpacking.

There are ways of finding water in the desert. But, if you hope to rely on them for basic drinking and cooking water, it would be best not to be too far from civilization. You can survive without water for two, maybe three days.

Water can be found in the pulp of certain types of cacti. The barrel cactus is one of the best. But the prickly pear cactus also contains enough moisture for emergencies. Break open the cactus. Scoop out the pulp inside and chew moisture from it. Do not eat the pulp.

Look for water under large rocks and boulders in a dry stream bed. When the water is flowing in these streams, it undermines rocks and causes deep holes on their downstream sides. The water in the depressions is shielded by the rocks, which helps retard evaporation.

In the desert as in the mountains, water runs to the lowest available level, which may be underground. Search for water at the base of hills, under rocky ledges and outcroppings, and in potholes. Dig for water in moist sand.

Potholes catch rainwater and act as natural reservoirs.

Basically they are depressions in rock formations and can be found anywhere in the rocky desert. Shaded ones retain water longer since they are shielded from the sun.

A body's daily demand for water varies. And different people drink varying amounts of water out of habit and training. Tennis players, for instance, usually require more water during a match than those engaged in a friendly chess game. Water intake depends on a person's metabolism as well as the amount of exertion involved. The temperature and humidity of the environment also are factors in determining the quantity of moisture needed.

The body loses liquid as well as salt through perspiration. At times when thirst is not satiated by drinking, the system may need salt. You can purchase salt tablets at drugstores. Or crystals of rock salt, purchased at supermarkets, can be used. One-fourth teaspoon of salt in a cup of water will satisfy the craving for liquids. The balance between salt and water in the body is complex and vital. Water is a major ingredient of the body, whereas salt assists in retaining it. With strenuous exercise, drink when thirsty and increase daily salt intake. This prevents dehydration and maintains the body at an optimal operating level.

WATER IN SNOW COUNTRY

In the wintertime, most water sources are buried beneath a thick layer of ice and snow. Some deep, swift-moving streams and ponds fed by warm springs can remain partially ice-free. However, through the action of frigid air meeting not-as-cold water, a fragile dome of ice generally forms, extending from the bank out towards the center of the water. In turn, snow piles up on this ledge, making it unstable. For these reasons, bending over the edge of a two-foot snowbank to scoop water into a container is risky. Very likely the bank will avalanche into the stream, bringing you with it. Instead, stand several feet away from the bank and obtain water by throwing a wide-mouthed plastic bottle attached to a twelve-foot nylon cord into the open water. Pull out the bottle, hand over hand and fill other containers from it.

Remember that below-freezing temperatures do not disinfect water. Once contaminated, it will remain so during the winter even if frozen into ice. Water unsafe to drink in the summer will make you just as sick in the winter.

Hiking in snow is like walking on water. The thirst-quenching substance is everywhere. Pick up a clump of fresh, white crystals and taste it. Too much snow can cause diarrhea and stomach discomfort. However, one clump of snow taken to alleviate thirst every hour or so will cause no digestive upset. Pluck a bunch of snow and plop it into the mouth to satisfy a craving for liquids. Try it. Experience the release from civilized restrictions. While water is an everyday phenomenon, utilizing snow for the body's needs is novel. Melt nature's nectar on the tongue, not just as an experiment, but to meet a definite need. It is a powerful reminder that water does not come from an intricate plumbing system but is captured by the earth's basin from the heavens. Droplets fall from the sky like so many tiny UFOs. Yet no fanfare accompanies the spectacle. It is taken for granted.

Melting snow into water is a time- and fuel-consuming chore. Heap a large pot with clean snow. Cover, and place on a stove or over an open fire. Pans can be scorched easily during the snow-thawing procedure; so check the process frequently. As the snow dissolves, add more. One pot of snow makes about one-third pot of water. New, powdery snow contains less moisture than old "corn" or crunch snow. Some wintertime camping buffs contend that snow-liquified water tastes "flat." They recommend infusing it with oxygen by passing it back and forth several times from pan to pot. This supposedly improves flavor according to water connoisseurs. However, in most cases, the water is not taken straight anyway, but mixed with instant chocolate or fruit drinks. Or it is used for a dehydrated, one-pot meal mix, like ham cheddarton. Water is not an end in itself then but a means of preparing nourishing, tasty drinks and meals.

PURIFYING WATER

Pure water cannot be identified by taste, smell, or sight. Only chemical analysis can differentiate safe water from contaminated. Of course, there are some common-sense methods. For instance, foul odor or floating debris warns the camper to beware. On the other hand, use water from an isolated stream, without any forms of pollution flowing into it upstream, without concern about its level of purity.

A wise outdoorsperson travels prepared to purify questionable water. An easy, effective method is to dissolve five Halazone tablets in one quart of water. Wait thirty minutes. The water is then ready to drink. Halazone may be purchased at most drugstores.

Boiling water for at least ten minutes is another way of disinfecting it. However, the boiling point of water decreases 1 degree centigrade for every 1,000-foot rise in elevation. At sea level, water is purified by 10 minutes of boiling, but it needs 15 minutes of boiling at 5,000 feet and 20 minutes at 8,000 feet.

Unless you spend a lot of time in the mountains, talking about elevation may seem meaningless, even confusing. But altitude directly affects hikers and it is important to know about. Driving from Cincinnati, Ohio with an elevation of 490 feet, for instance, to Cheyenne, Wyoming, that stands 6,100 feet above sea level, a person ascends 5,610 feet. Cheyenne is located in the middle of a sagebrush prairie with the closest mountain range, the Medicine Bow peaks, about 85 miles west. But altitude-wise it is a lofty town, higher in fact, than the mile-high city of Denver.

With such an increase of altitude, breathing becomes more difficult. Exercise seems more strenuous. Movement is an effort. Of course, the body adjusts to altitude after a few days. But initially, the increased elevation above sea level is a shock to the body. Similar to jet lag, altitude lag should be taken into account when planning a camping trip in a section of country much higher or lower in elevation than where you live. Set aside a day or two to relax once you reach the trailhead before starting out on a strenuous expedition.

The process of boiling water demands time and fuel. Halazone tablets, on the other hand, are more economical. They purify water without the waste of a limited fuel supply. Costing between two and three cents per tablet, they take up little room in a pack and are handy and convenient.

From a survival standpoint, there are many ingenious ways of obtaining water. These methods are for the ill-prepared camper or persons in a life-and-death struggle with nature as a result of a natural disaster. Bradford Angier is an author who specializes in survival techniques. His books deal with how a person can rely on her wits to live off the country. While interesting and entertaining, Angier's works give information that might prove to be a lifesaver some day. His *Living off the Country* (Stackpole Books, Seventh Printing, 1968), for instance, describes how to build a solar still to obtain water. Fundamentally, this can be used in either the desert or in the snow when fuel is too limited to use for melting snow in a pot.

LAUNDRY

On a trip shorter than two weeks, washing clothes is an extravagant chore. Because you wash clothes every Monday at home is not a valid reason for following the same routine in the wilderness. Of course, the necessity for doing laundry rests with several factors. For example, how many changes of clothes did you bring? Are the clothes actually dirty and saturated with perspiration? How do you feel about wearing the same pair of jeans for one week?

Packing one extra pair of slacks and two additional shirts can virtually eliminate thoughts of having to take time to do laundry during a two-week jaunt. However, underwear and socks may require daily soaking and rinsing. Unless you are bosomy and need the support, omit the bra. If you feel comfortable without one, leave it at home. It is one less piece of clothing to dirty and launder. In this way, the laundry problem is simplified to panties and wool socks.

Woolite is a cold water detergent, containing no phosphates (a dangerous stream pollutant). It is biodegradable and soaks items clean in three minutes. No rubbing. Fill a plastic basin with available water. It need not be pure or warm. Add a capful of Woolite. Swish to make suds and add clothes. Soak for three minutes. Squeeze excess moisture from the clothes. Pour the sudsy water over the ground. Rinse the articles thoroughly by refilling the basin and dipping the clothes in and out of the water until no more suds appear.

Drying Clothes

According to Woolite directions, do not hang the clothes in the sun. Instead, drape them over shaded branches of a tree or bush. Or spread them over the sunless part of a rock. A gentle breeze will dry clothing quickly.

Time your laundering chores so that items will be dry by evening. At dusk, if the clothes are still damp (wool socks dry very slowly), bring them inside the tent where they will not be saturated by dew. Hang them over an available pole or rig a makeshift clothesline inside the tent.

In below-freezing temperatures, some hardy folk "dry" wet clothes by allowing them to freeze and then shake out the ice crystals. No matter how hard the garments are shook, however, a few ice crystals always seem to stay behind. It is a chilling experience to put them on once again.

On cold days and nights, it is more effective to remove moisture from clothes by means of a fire. Hang them on a long stick and place the clothes close enough to the fire to dry out, but not so close that they scorch. The heat from a campfire evaporates moisture from wet items, even wool socks, in a relatively short period of time.

How to Make Your Own Soap

Even heavy cotton slacks can be washed in a small pail of water with Woolite. But many backwoodswomen, who have spent weeks in the wilderness, heat water in a large cook pot. They add hot water detergent and the soiled garments. Especially stalwart women pride themselves on the fact that they even make their own soap while afield. They pour scalding water several times over campfire ashes and use the resulting liquid in wash water. In fact, pioneer women had no other type of soap. Ashes from the kitchen stove were recycled by pouring hot water over them and draining. Through this process of leaching, lye—largely

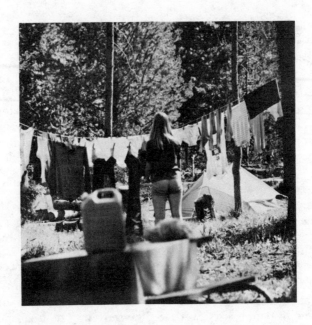

Laundry is time-, water-, and energy-consuming. This chore is unnecessary on trips shorter than two weeks.

potash—was produced and later used as a cleansing
substance.

Using a large stick, stripped of bark, agitate the clothes
to loosen and wash away dirt. Do not soak them because
of the possibility of colors fading and shrinkage. Rinse in
warm water, constantly stirring to remove soap. Wring out
the clothes and hang in the sun. The combination of sun
and wind facilitates evaporation of moisture. Drying heavy
jeans in this manner does make them stiff, but at least they
are clean. Cotton blouses may be washed in this manner
or by Woolite. Of course, rags used as an emergency re-
placement for sanitary napkins should be soaked and

washed in hot, sudsy water and laid flat in the sun, on high grass or bushes, so they can be bleached.

The best time to launder is when you have found a suitable place to bathe or shower (see Chapter 7). A few, daring people swim with their clothes on, disrobe in the pond, and spread the garments out on a nearby limb or boulder. Soap is not involved in washing either themselves or their clothes. Instead, the movement of swimming dislodges most dirt. The idea of needing soap to wash bodies and apparel to a faultless shine is largely psychological. Of course, the need for soap depends on the extent the item is soiled.

DISHWASHING

Surprising as it may sound, dishwashing can be nearly eliminated while camping. It depends on planning and altering the stringent habits of spotlessness to which most modern women adhere. First, decide you will eat off paper plates. Yes, paper plates are flimsy. But presently on the market are small, basketlike holders for paper plates that give backbone and support. They do not require washing since the food is placed on the paper plate. But they allow a camper to hold the plate in one hand and a fork in the other. There is no fear that the paper plate will suddenly fold, spilling an entire meal all over the feaster's lap.

Paper cups are usually crushed in a food bag or in a pack. A metal or heavy-duty plastic cup, with a handle that can hook onto the hiker's belt loop, is handy. It can double as a bowl and can be rinsed clean with plain water. Then it can be replaced on the belt and allowed to drip-dry.

Silverware, on the other hand, is indispensable. Plastic eating utensils are susceptible to breakage and are not tough enough to withstand the rugged demands of outdoor use. Plastic forks cannot spear meatballs. The knives cannot cut adequately and the spoons melt in hot coffee. It is sensible to pack along a stainless steel fork and spoon. A pocketknife can replace the dinner knife.

As strange as it might seem, cooking pots and utensils are not washed with soap and water. In the outdoor camp kitchen, mounds of soap complicate cleaning chores and are not necessary. In fact, soap residue can be harmful. It can touch off a bad case of diarrhea. Ordinarily rinse water is not in abundance and soapy dishes are not adequately rinsed.

Boiling water, not soap, kills bacteria on pans and utensils. Suds loosen dirt and food particles and break down grease to hasten cleaning. But bacteria remains. Only boiling water destroys "germs." In fact, if eating and cooking utensils are smothered in boiling water, suds are uncalled for and actually wasteful if the water supply is limited.

After plates are heaped with beef Stroganoff or lasagne, fill the cook pot with boiling water. During dinner, the steaming water acts to disengage stuck-on food. After supper, dig a small hole with the boot heel and deposit the waste water from the pot. Cover the cavity with soil and pack down. Pour more boiling water into the kettle and give a final rinsing. Douse silverware with boiling water and rub clean with a paper towel. Be sure to remove all food residue, especially that caked in between the prongs of forks. That is the extent of the dishwashing chores.

The tools for maintaining a clean camp are a pot of boiling water and several rolls of paper towels. Used toweling is burned in the campfire. Boiling water is the first line of defense, disarming potentially harmful substances. Paper towels do the rest, removing food specks and grease. Old timers substituted stream and pond moss for paper towels.

Yes, this procedure differs greatly from the dishwashing routine at home. But it is quick, easy, and effectively cleans pots and utensils. It fits right into the outdoor scene; it gets the job done with basic tools and minimum amount of work.

Soaking may be mandatory, especially when a thick layer of cooked-on food lines the pot. For burned-on food, boil water in the pot on the stove or over the fire, simultaneously scraping the pot clean with a wooden spoon. The action of water boiling agitates most scorched particles free from the pot. Prevention, however, is the best way to solve cleaning problems. For example, food is not as likely to stick to Teflon-coated camp pots and pans. Cooking meals over low heat or glowing coals and frequent stirring likewise ensures flavorful dishes without food being burned on.

GARBAGE

Garbage and commercial development are major destroyers of wilderness. Once they gain a foothold in an area, they run rampant and take over. Primitive people have few worldly possessions and no garbage. They recycle everything. A tin can is treasured, saved, and used as a drinking cup. A sheet of newspaper is twisted into a cone-shape and serves as a paper bag. In it, simple people carry eggs, string beans, or cherries which they purchase from the local market. Some of them "paper" their houses with it for insulation. There is a touch of ingenuity in their ability to find a use for almost anything that North Americans classify as useless garbage. Upon entering the wilderness, outdoorspeople should adopt the attitude that there is no such thing as garbage. A moment of perceptive thinking can discover the value of even the simplest item.

Organized campgrounds provide trash cans at campsites. Deposit nonburnable refuse, such as bottles, jars, cans, and chicken bones in the can. At a few campgrounds, underground garbage disposals are also available. These do away with eggshells, grease, potato peelings, and stale salads, which attract scavenging animals and birds and can eventually emit offensive odors. At camp, keep scraps in one plastic bag and feed the disposal each day's supply before bedtime. Grease can be a problem. Some campers store grease in an empty shortening can with a plastic, tight-fitting lid. They reuse it for such dishes as pan-fried fish, chicken, or pot roast. Others sprinkle bacon grease in with the dog's food. Canine lovers say that it gives the dog's coat a healthy sheen. A few funnel the grease into an empty can and let it coagulate before they toss it into the garbage pail. Eating dehydrated food eliminates the need for grease for shortening, and then it is a problem no longer.

When in the wilderness, burn food scraps. Pour dish water and grease into a hole about four to six inches deep and cover with soil. Burying garbage is not a good idea since animals will dig it up and scatter what they do not eat. Pack unburnable trash out with you in plastic bags. For all practical purposes, aluminum foil does not burn in a campfire. But it is convenient and versatile for cooking purposes.

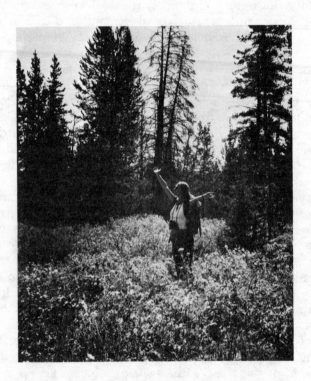

Without leaving a trace of your presence behind, you are as clean and refreshing as the outdoors.

Fold the used foil into a tiny packet and return it to your backpack. With the rest of the unburnables, carry it back to civilization with you.

Burying garbage in snow is a sneaky way of littering. When the snow melts, the pile of garbage stays. Do not hide trash in snow because, come spring, it will be exposed as litter.

Cleanliness is important and can be achieved by follow-

ing common-sense principles. Burn garbage if you can. If
not, carry it with you in a heavy-duty, plastic bag. A number of outdoorswomen plan their trip so all they have to
carry out as trash is a few, folded squares of used aluminum
foil. Along the homebound trail, they may come across beer
cans, pop tops, or crunched up pieces of foil. Dedicated,
self-sacrificing woodswomen carry out the garbage left
behind by the careless. This is the ultimate: cleaning up
after someone else. But until more people realize the harm
they cause by scattering empty containers over the wilderness, this is exactly what thoughtful people will have to do.

10

Outdoor Hobbies

The mind can be puzzling. It can exclude the real and paint an imaginary but lovely world. It can remind you of shameful deeds that happened decades ago and that you assumed had been long forgotten. Many people feel victimized by remembrances that seem to intrude on the present. Others prefer to meditate on the past, abandoning the here-and-now to pass unnoticed. A large number of persons, however, do not realize that they have control over their thoughts. It may take practice. Chronic day-dreamers require determination to jolt them back into the present. Worriers predictably imagine and expect the worst. They need to reprimand and force themselves to think only good things.

But the best way to exercise control over the mind is to perform an interesting, attention-consuming task. An enjoyable activity is the best defense against boredom. The body —not merely the mind—can be active and live a little. Having fun opens a mental hatch, allowing you to climb out of yourself. Concentrate on hitting a tennis ball over the net or bicycling without holding onto the handlebars and forget yourself. Occupy the mind with a goal outside yourself. As a result, you will be less critical of yourself and others, more interested and interesting.

To a family-oriented woman, home, children, and husband are extensions of herself. Leave them behind and go out into the outdoors. Find your true self. Not by actively searching but by engrossing yourself in an aspect of nature. First, however, you need to become acquainted with an outdoor activity or hobby that appeals to you. Cultivate a pleasurable skill. It will reward you with a lifetime of fun and a reliable way of finding refuge from yourself.

Two hobbies that develop an acute awareness of nature as well as offer years of exploration and discovery are outdoor photography and rock hunting.

OUTDOOR PHOTOGRAPHY

"Outdoor photography" has an ominous ring to it. It sounds too serious, mysterious, complicated for the average person who basically just wants to have a good time. But on the contrary, outdoor photography is simple. It involves recording on film what appears especially beautiful or breathtaking to the eyes. The guiding principle is always carry your camera within easy reach.

The camera you own now is the right one to begin with. Self-satisfying photography does not start with fancy equipment. Rather, penetrating observation, the "photographic eye," is the key to outstanding picture-taking. The art of recording nature through the camera lens can be a neverending process of development. It is a new way of looking at the surroundings. You catch yourself commenting, "That would make a great photo."

Always bring your camera. Then there is no excuse for missing a potentially powerful shot. Walking along a familiar path, for example, you find a mallard duck's nest with seven freckled, white eggs beside a cottonwood tree. You have passed this way many times before. But this time, there are the makings of a memorable photo.

The camera belongs on a strap around the neck. Then, when you catch a glimpse of a spotted deer fawn nursing,

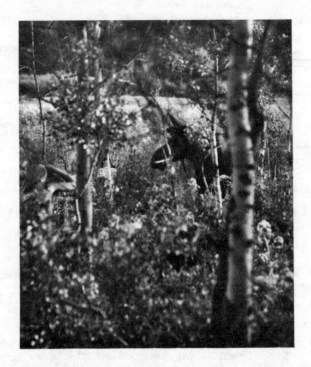

The key to successful outdoor photography is: bring your camera every-where. Here a photographer is getting too close to a moose.

your camera is handy to capture the unexpected. An action picture tells a story while a still life records. Storing the camera away in a rucksack limits you to scenics and flowers. Unpredictable animals and birds will not pose while you disengage the camera from the confining pack.

Photographing Wild Animals

Eventually photography becomes a habit and you begin to notice fine, meaningful detail. A gnawed tip of a willow bush says that a big game animal has been browsing here. A jagged hole as round as a tennis ball, bored into a dying tree, announces the presence of a nesting pair of wood-peckers. A pile of empty freshwater clam shells beside a stream tells the tale of the gluttonous mink.

How to Get Close to Animals. Where wildlife leaves signs—tracks, droppings, trees stripped of bark—the pho-tographer should patiently wait. Hide behind a bush or other natural blind with camera focused, cocked, and ready to shoot. Animals follow a daily, seasonal routine. Where they have once been, they will return unless threat of danger forces them outside the boundaries of their territory. Exer-cise patience and slowly work your way within shooting distance.

Capturing wild animals on film is a matter of wits. The photographer needs to be thoroughly familiar with the ani-mal's habitat and habits. She must fool the animal on his own ground. Wild creatures are shy. They associate humans with danger and try to avoid them at all costs. The photog-rapher acts so as to convince the deer or woodpecker that she is not human but another type of wild creature. Motion-less, she is also silent except for the click of the shutter open-ing and closing. Animals are observant and curious. You want them to lower their defensive guard and examine this strange being, namely you, at closer range.

Camouflage clothes—the green and brown-spotted jacket and loose-fitting olive drab slacks characteristic of the mili-tary—help the photographer blend in with the natural vegetation. Your outline is not as readily decipherable as it would be with bright clothes. Animals adjust rather quickly to the presence of a tent also. The photographer sets up the camera inside with the lens extending through a hole in the tent. Birds and animals become accustomed to the structure and behave naturally. Sage grouse, for instance, perform elaborate mating rituals in the spring, even if a camouflage tent is set up in the middle of the strutting grounds.

Whether or not you want to go to great lengths to obtain outstanding wildlife photos, it is good to know that these measures are available and have been proven effective. With an Instamatic or other relatively inexpensive camera, the photographer needs to position herself at least twenty-five to fifty feet from the animal to guarantee good photos.

Photographing Insects

Outdoor photography increases powers of observation, practical knowledge of wildlife, and the understanding of what it takes to get close to birds and animals. However, it also directs attention to the small things in nature—for instance, butterflies and moths, that often go unnoticed. You are sitting beside a wild rose bush next to a frequently traveled game trail. Visions of a doe deer in her summer coat of sable brown fill your thoughts. Then your attention is diverted to a colony of funny-looking, odd-acting beetles. You wonder what their world is like; what they are doing and why.

Entomology is a branch of zoology that deals exclusively with the study of insects. In North America, excluding Mexico, 88,600 species of insects have been catalogued by entomologists. Species of insects outnumber birds by more than 100 to 1. While housewives and farmers associate insects with creepy, crawly pests that eat crops, plants, flowers, clothes, and wood, most insects benefit the natural environment. The pollinating services rendered are worth more than any damage they may do. Insects occur almost everywhere (except in the ocean) and make up more than half of all living organisms on earth. They cannot be all bad.

Insects are small and docile enough to be caught and examined in the hand. However, certain characteristics are so tiny that a hand lens may be useful in pinpointing the finer details. First, inspect the size, shape, and color of the insect. The general appearance places it in an order. Then, the individual parts of the insect—the antennae, legs, bristles, wings, etc.—distinguish it as belonging to a specific family.

A *Field Guide to Insects* by Donald J. Borror and Richard E. White (Houghton Mifflin Co., 1970) describes in detail how to collect, preserve, and identify 579 families of insects. Color plates and diagrams facilitate identification for the beginner.

There is more to the insect world than learning names,

families, and orders. And photography is the medium through which you learn about it. The possibility of snapping an exceptional photo justifies a person's sitting in one location for an entire day. During that time, a microcosm with the insect as the prime mover unfolds. While sitting on a folding stool in a marsh, not far from a small, shallow pond, you wait for a pair of sandhill cranes to arrive on the scene for their unruly spring mating dance. In the meantime, you notice that the air is full of insects that fly up and down—vertically, rather than horizontally. They land on your camera, nose, leg, any available spot. They rest awhile and then begin their enchanting, hypnotizing, bouncing bobbing again. Fragile creatures, they seem to have no function other than being light, airy, and full of spunk. The messengers of spring, acting out nature's mood. Where do they come from?

Gazing into the glistening surface of the pond, you recognize similar creatures riding the ripples. They seem to emerge from the water. There they sit, rapidly beating their wings free of moisture. Suddenly, like miniature helicopters, they lift off, completely different-looking organisms from the ones that first appeared out of the depths of the pond. A fish thrashes from the water trying to gulp down the tasty insects—too late.

Swirls on the water surface indicate that fish favor these dancing flies as food. The wings work frantically. Some of the delicate ones are sucked into hungry stomachs. Others make their escape above the surface. And they dance so enticingly two or three feet above the ravenous creatures below.

The insects are mayflies. The drama is their transformation from nymphs to adults. Occurring quietly, without ado, the process would have passed unnoticed without comment, if you had not been there.

Adult mayflies live a day, maybe two, and do not feed. Their prime functions are mating and being food for fish. Fly fishers use imitation mayflies quite often to fool fish, especially trout.

Photography freezes the moment, stops the action, and records it on film. Through prints or slides you can relive each step of the nature walk, backpack trip, or fishing extravaganza. The camera can be a faithful recorder or it can be the vehicle for self-expression. You sense a special feeling about a scene or situation and try to convey the mood through the photo. Like a painting, the creative photo communicates a universal principle, emotion, or lesson. The essence of this miracle of the camera resides within the photographer. However, certain techniques can be followed to assist the artist with the masterpiece.

Photographic Techniques

Techniques are important once you have mastered the basics. Hold the camera steady and straight while shooting a picture. Choose the right exposure. Make sure the photo includes essential elements. For instance, when you are snapping pictures of a prairie dog standing outside his den, do not cut off any part of him. After these principles are second nature, then concern yourself about techniques.

How to Compose a Picture. A technique is the way you construct a picture to attract the eye of the viewer to a focal point and the central message. Framing is one way to do this. It involves placing a natural object, such as tree, boulder, bush, or driftwood, in the foreground of the photo to add definition and depth. The eye is accustomed to looking out onto the world from a frame, that is, the face. The eyes are used to seeing your own nose in the middle of every scene. Such a frame is needed in photos to give them depth. A photo of a wide expanse of landscape, for example, is uninteresting to the casual viewer. There is nothing to focus on. Just uninterrupted land. Include a nearby tree as a border and the viewer feels that she is right there absorbing the scenery.

Lighting. Early morning sunlight and the light just before sunset lend golden glow to photos. Camera results at these prime shooting times appear to be sparked by the sun. Tones and shadows are especially attractive and pleasing to the eye.

For most photos of people and animals when pure recording is the goal, you will want the subject evenly illuminated. Position people facing or angled to the sun so you can naturally light up their faces. (When doing this be careful of the sun casting the photographer's shadow into the photo. Unless you are wary of the "phantom shadow," it can easily slip into the picture and ruin the effect you are trying to achieve.) But for the "arty" or "moody" photos, where mood or illusion is paramount, shoot when the sun is behind or slightly angled from the subject. Back-lit photos emphasize the texture and silhouette of the subject. A squirrel, for instance, appears as a ball of fur; the sun outlines each hair, making an unusual, spectacular photo of a common squirrel.

Side-lit shots cast light and shadows in varying degrees on the subject and produce interesting contrasts. A side-lit photo of a frog, for example, emphasizes the glistening eye and the "slippery" skin.

Bad weather can add a lifelike dimension to a photo. Rain, heavy clouds, and snow suggest dampness, dreariness, and hardship. The power and strength of nature comes through. Weather in action. Most photographers pack their cameras away in foul weather, but that is the time to come up with truly unique photos.

Plan the picture. Keep photos simple. Including too much in one picture results in cluttering. The eye is not directed to a central point and feels confused and puzzled. Place the featured subject off center a bit. In a photo of a chipmunk running across a log, the animal should be off-center. He should be scampering towards open space and not right "out" of the photo. In other words, give your subjects "running room."

Change camera positions. Shoot from above, in a tree or on a hill. Or capture your subjects on ground level from the stomach position. An unusual angle gives an added twist to an ordinary setting, increasing the attractiveness of the photo. The more you change camera angles and positions, the better your pictures will be.

Books on Photography

Photographing Nature, a complete volume of the *Life* Library of Photography (Time, Inc., 1971), details photographic techniques, including those used for underwater photography. The beautiful illustrations inspire the outdoor photographer regardless of the level of expertise. Specific information describes how different effects can be achieved.

Also to be recommended is *Camera Afield* by Sid Latham (Stackpole, 1976). Latham, one of the original lensmen of *Life* magazine, not only shares his photographic expertise with the reader but also offers invaluable tips about protecting cameras and film from such travel hazards as x-ray inspections of luggage at airports and extreme climatic conditions.

Photographic Equipment

The camera you presently own is the means of determining whether outdoor photography is for you. Every time you venture outdoors—even for a picnic lunch—bring along your camera. Concentrate on recording the outdoors as you see it through your own eyes. Your photos can help others value nature as much as you do. Photography is more than gathering aunts, uncles, and cousins together for a group picture. But it is up to you to give your pictures that little extra that distinguishes them from snapshots. Through imagination, creativity, and ingenuity, you can become an expert in the photographic message.

Cameras and Lenses. If photography appeals to you, the question of more and better equipment will undoubtedly arise. Telephoto lenses act as binoculars or a telescope in bringing distant objects up close. They magnify so the photographer can shoot a large image without moving too close to the subject. These lenses simplify wildlife photography. Stalking is not as critical. A good photo can be snapped from fifty yards away. A 200mm lens is a versatile telephoto lens and is not too expensive.

However, a major drawback in utilizing telephoto lenses

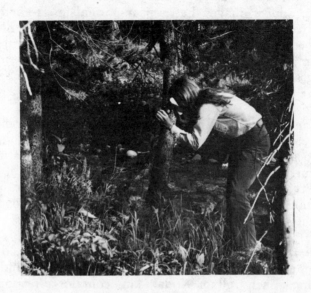

A 200-mm lens enables you to get a close-up of an animal without venturing too close.

is that they require a camera body that can take more than one lens. The most popular type is the 35mm, single-lens reflex (SLR) camera. In contrast to the range finder camera, the SLR enables the photographer to compose the picture through the same lens that takes it. This facilitates quick, easy picture snapping.

SLR 35s are relatively small, lightweight, and convenient to carry wherever you go; but, they are not cheap. The cost begins at $200. Before making such an investment, be certain you will use the camera often enough to make it worth the price. Used cameras and lenses are available at camera stores at reasonable prices. From the general appearance and condition of the camera and lens, judge for yourself whether it is in adequate shape. Reputable photo stores, provided they know you, will permit you to take a used camera out and shoot some film through it before purchase. This is the best way to check out a used camera.

A normal lens for a 35mm camera is the 55mm. This lens produces images that appear normal in size and perspective to the eye. For the outdoor photographer, this lens is not as useful as the 200mm. The wide-angle lens—21mm, 28mm, or 35mm—gives a wider view and smaller images than the eye sees. It is especially effective for scenics where an entire mountain range can be included in a single photo.

Many name-brand cameras and lenses are on the market today. Honeywell Pentax, Canon, Nikon, Minolta, and Leica are top camera manufacturers, and each features a system of lenses. Their workmanship is usually of high quality, thus insuring years of faithful service. Because of this, a used camera with a telephoto lens can be a good buy for the novice.

Film. Coordinating the type of film and film speed with the operation of the camera can be complicated and perplexing. Each roll of Kodak film contains directions on recommended exposure settings. These are helpful. But for the newcomer, individual instruction may be necessary until you get the hang of it.

Manufacturers describe their film by its sensitivity to light or speed, as indicated by its ASA rating. ASA, or the American Standards Association, grades film according to the amount of light needed to produce a normal image. The higher the ASA rating, the more sensitive the film is to light, requiring less illumination than lower ASA ratings. Slow films range from an ASA of 20 to 50; medium speeds from 100 to 200, and fast films from 400 to 1250. A light meter operates in conjunction with the ASA setting of the film.

Film, of course, may be black and white or color. The development process of black and white film is less expensive than it is for color. It is smart to practice techniques and new ideas with black and white film. Also black and white is more economical to shoot when you are familiarizing yourself with a new camera or lens.

Color film produces either prints or slides. When the

name of the film ends in "color" (for example, Kodacolor), prints are the end result. When "chrome" is the suffix (for instance, Kodachrome), the film produces slides. The operating instructions that accompany each camera generally recommend the broad category of film type. But the decision of slides or prints is up to the photographer.

Outdoor photography is full of adventure. Outdoors, equipped with camera and plenty of film, you can preserve your discoveries and experiences. Enjoy them over and over again. Compared to the results, film is inexpensive. Do not sell yourself short by limiting photography to only one or two rolls a day. Bring along plenty of reinforcements. Nature is unlimited and so are the opportunities.

ROCK HUNTING

The rockhound tradition is a bloodline descendant of the prospector who scoured the rocky terrain of the frontier during the 1800s. The motivation is different. The rock hunter does not seek a fortune, in terms of what gold can buy. Modern travel by dune buggy, trail bike, car, or airplane places the rockhound in rich mineral fields for a day, weekend, or vacation. Today's prospector is not forced to disavow family, friends, and society to live alone in the rocky wilderness with a faithful mule. But the undying belief that tomorrow will uncover a priceless find is the same. The exciting mystery—the possibility of a valuable stone lying buried at your feet—is ever present.

Rock hunting is an increasingly popular sport. Clubs and societies are in existence all over the country. A group of gem or mineral seekers shares experiences. Where one rough piece of jade or agate is found, others are bound to be. Several searchers can cover more ground faster and more efficiently than a lone person can. Who knows, maybe other valuable minerals may be discovered in the process. Rock hunters pool their resources for enthusiastic digs and to interest others in the adventuresome, satisfying sport of rock hunting.

Rock hunting is a misnomer, perhaps an understatement. It does not mean shuffling around in a mound of gravel,

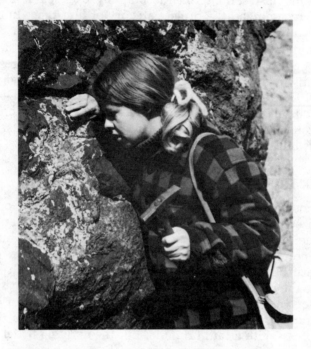

Rock hunting is an increasingly popular outdoor sport.

making mud pies, or digging holes indiscriminately. Based on knowledge and experience—and tips from practiced colleagues—it is an intelligent search for rocks that on closer inspection contain fossils, gems, or prized minerals. Here geology and archaeology are within reach of the average person. Within your grasp lies the story of the earth's formation. The fiercesome processes of wind, water, glacier, and volcano scraped, chipped, reduced, altered what existed and made something different. Every physical phenomenon is recorded within the rocks and minerals that make up the earth. To learn about pre-man history, read the earth's crust.

Fossils

A fossil is one of the sought-after finds of rockhounds. It is a trace of a living organism from a previous geological period, indelibly marked in a rock or on the earth's crust. To find and identify a fossil is an unforgettable experience. By sparking your imagination, it acts like a time machine. You transport yourself back in time thousands of years and speculate how it must have been with huge reptiles, like the dinosaurs, roaming the earth's surface.

A fossil can be the actual preserved remains of a mammoth animal. Of course, this type is extremely rare. More plentiful, petrified wood is a type of fossil in which the original organism has been replaced by mineral. A mold, however, is the most common kind of fossil. It consists of the impression of a plant, animal, or fish in soft mud. After the body decayed, the impression remained, permanently preserved. An outline of a plant, the footprints of a tyrannosaurus, a cavity formed by a shell—concrete proof of life that existed before man. From them, geologists learn the age of the rock strata in which they are found. In addition, conditions of the atmosphere in which they lived can be pinpointed. Was it dry or moist, cold or hot? Was the water fresh or salty?

However, a rock is just a useless hunk of stone unless you know a few facts about minerals, gems, or fossils. A rock with an insectlike design imprinted on it is not a coincidence or a haphazard quirk of nature. It is a fossil. By critically

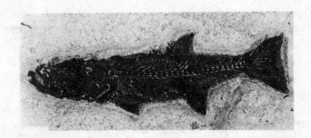

This is a fossil fish from Fossil Buttes near Kemmerer, Wyoming.

examining a simple, gray, dull-looking rock, a wealth of knowledge may be gained. This revelation is what changes a nonchalant rock kicker into a fanatic rock hunter.

Mineral Composition of Rocks

Rocks and minerals are the most plentiful and unevenly distributed substances known. Rocks are natural formations, making up the earth's outer layer, composed mainly of minerals. Minerals are natural substances with a definite chemical composition but are neither animal nor vegetable. Rock-forming minerals contain eight or ten chemicals in various combinations. These are oxygen, silicon, aluminum, iron, calcium, magnesium, sodium, potassium, sulphur, and carbon.

Types of Rock

There are three different types of rock: igneous, sedimentary, and metamorphic. Igneous rocks, for instance, were formed from cooling of molten lava. Small crystals in rocks were cooled at or near the surface of the earth while the larger crystals cooled slowly below the surface. Mineral particles then became interlocked. Granite is one of the most common igneous rocks.

Granite is composed of quartz, feldspar, mica, and occasionally hornblende. Quartz can be identified by its glassy luster and its hard texture; it cannot be scratched with a knife and cuts glass. Quartz is one of the most abundant materials in the crust of the earth. Besides being an important part of granite, it is the chief material of most sand and sandstone and can be found in lavas and gneiss. As crystals, it ornaments the walls of cavities in rocks and forms veins. Other minerals are often deposited at the same time and in this way the ores of the precious metals are often associated with quartz.

Crystalline quartz comes in many different colors, forming a wide selection of gems. If quartz is colorless and has transparent crystals, it is called rock crystal—a believable imitation of the diamond and a semiprecious stone in its own right. If quartz is purple, it is called amethyst, a semi-precious stone. When quartz is glassy white, but not transparent, it is milky quartz. If it is bright red, it is carnelian; if brownish red, sard; if banded in various colors, agate. Jasper is dull red or brown quartz. Bloodstone is green with red spots. All of these can make attractive, unusual jewelry. Consider amethysts, agate, and rock crystals hiding in a stone, waiting to be chiseled to freedom by you. And there are many other varieties of gems and minerals besides.

Flint is smoky or gray quartz with small, shell-like fractures. The Petrified Forest National Park in eastern Arizona is a natural wonder and demonstrates how flint evolves. Great trees were changed to agate and flint by silica, the substance of quartz, permeating the plant tissue so that the texture of the wood was preserved.

Before matches were invented and mass-produced, flint was more important to a family than a horse. Striking flint

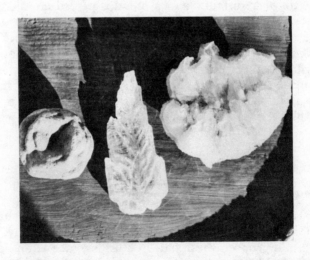

Triangular specimen is petrified wood. The rest of the rocks are various types of agate.

with steel produced sparks. By directing sparks to very dry tinder, a small fire was ignited. With loving care, the tiny flame was nourished with kindling and bigger branches were added until it became a respectable, warmth-producing blaze.

Indians used flint for arrowheads and hatchets. These can be discovered scattered throughout the Midwest and the western United States. Early Indians returned each year to a special location to renew their flint supplies. One traditional location was along the Wind River in Wyoming. Here large quantities of flint were discovered and considered sacred. Tribes would leave behind their used, chipped flint products and shape and sharpen new ones. The rockhound that stumbles across such an area will uncover invaluable relics of early man.

Rock hunting is a democratic sport. Simply walk at a slow pace through rocky terrain. Stop once in awhile at an intriguing rock formation and chip away with the prospector's pick and chisel. Start locally, in the backyard or city park. Pick up an appealing rock. Examine it: note color, luster, hardness, surface irregularities, crystalline structure. If the tip of a knifeblade or a chisel is placed on one of the surface cracks and tapped with a hammer, the mineral will break open without shattering. The inside of the rock may be completely different from the exterior. The outside may be uninteresting, lifeless. A geode is a perfect example. On the surface, it looks ragged and worthless. Break it in half with a chisel and hammer. Inside is a fantasia of crystals with glittering, shimmering, and hypnotizing color.

Where to Spot Rock Trophies

Rock trophies can be spotted in areas of geological change. Erosion and landslides expose rocks that previously were deep underground. Fresh cuts in hillsides, excavation, quarries, and old mine dumps are prime locations for productive rock pursuits.

Rock Hunting Equipment

Besides pick, chisel, and pocketknife, handy rockhound gear includes a steel file, a small magnet, a magnifying glass, and a streak plate for testing. A streak plate is a piece of unglazed porcelain. When a mineral is rubbed across the surface of the plate, it leaves a fine powder that may be of a color entirely different from the mineral itself. Determining the "streak" of a mineral assists in properly identifying it. For further information and specifics about identifying minerals, read *The Rock-Hunter's Field Manual* by D. K. Fritzen (Harper and Brothers Publishers, 1959).

Guides to Rock Hunting Localities

Nearly every state, including Hawaii and Alaska, offers opportunities for seeking a prized rock, mineral, or natural gem. State travel commissions or tourist departments, headquartered in the capital city of each state, can provide information about rock hunters' clubs and can pinpoint sections of the state with reputations for enjoyable rock hunts. With a few leads from the travel commission, choose prime rock hunting cities. Write to the chamber of commerce of each. They will send booklets on rock hunting in their areas. Information will also be provided on the types of rocks and gems found locally, as well as the laws governing the collecting of petrified wood or searching for rocks on private and public lands.

A large number of rock hunters' organizations also supply maps of especially productive localities. They detail how to get there and what you will probably find, as well as where the nearest rock shops are situated.

In Kansas, for example, the Geological Survey located at the University of Kansas, Lawrence, Kansas 66044, puts out an excellent booklet entitled *Kansas Rocks and Minerals*. It discloses everything the beginner rock hunter needs to know. For the Appalachian area, a worthwhile resource book is *Appalachian Mineral and Gem Trails* by June Culp

Zeitner (available from Lapidary Journal, Inc., P.O. Box 2369, San Diego, California 92112 for $3.95).

New Hampshire is nicknamed the Granite State, and the state geologist recommends *The Geology of New Hampshire, Part III, Minerals and Mines* for those interested in learning more about the rock hunting potential there. For $1.50, the pamphlet can be obtained from the Division of Economic Development (P.O. Box 856, Concord, New Hampshire 03301).

A comprehensive guide to rock locations is the *Western Gem Hunters Atlas* by Cy Johnson (write to Cy Johnson, Box 288, Susanville, California 96130).

The list goes on. Each state offers something special to the rockhound. Go ahead. Pick up a piece of history. Look it over and place it in its proper place in the scheme of creation of the world. Identify and place it in your collection of the segments of the earth that you learned firsthand, on your own.

11

Fishing

The sport of fishing is nearly as old as the human race. At first, fish were sought as tasty, nourishing food, especially when game was scarce and berries, nuts, and plants were not yet ripe for gathering. Eventually, fish were esteemed as wary competitors. Young braves convinced the tribe of their guile and skill by fooling fish. They carved hooks from deer bone and attached them to a line and pole. But the ultimate test of man's superiority over fish was determining, and then catching, bait that fish would gulp without hesitation. Secondly, the bait, threaded onto a hook, was presented in a manner natural enough to attract fish. The complete process revolved around the ingenuity of the fisher. Because the primitive man designed and constructed his own equipment, fishing results directly reflected personal expertise.

Over thousands of years, fish have not changed much. Some anglers swear they get smarter every year. And they do stage the same thrilling battle for the modern fishermen as they did for the primitives. Fish still eat aquatic insects and fishers are still experimenting with bait to trick fish on

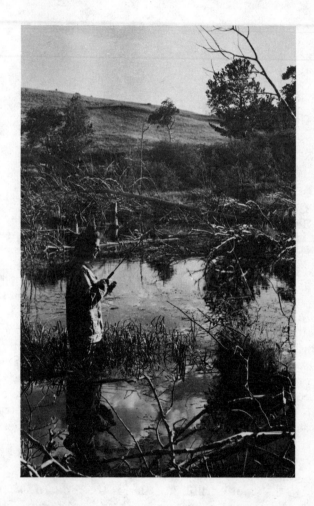

Thinking like a fish demands patience and practice, which can make women outstanding fishers.

a predictable basis. Today fish live in most streams, rivers, lakes, and ponds and can be depended on to give the clever angler—who can be you—a contest.

Traditionally, fishing has been considered a man's sport. However, women who have ventured into angling have discovered they are better equipped than many men for sharpening the sport into a skill. Patience is the virtue which transforms the angler into an artist. Outstanding fisherpeople display the amazing ability to think like a fish. When the hook has gone strikeless and fishless for thirty minutes or more, the fisher asks herself, "On a rainy, dreary day like today, where would I go if I were a rainbow trout?"

Know the basic habits and likes of the fish you are after and increase the simple pleasure of fishing. Besides being exciting and full of action, angling offers a delicious bonus —a wild feast of roasted fish.

Even though schools are available to teach specific fishing methods (see Chapter 1), the secrets of fishing can be learned by watching and asking questions of good fishers. Arrive at a local stream naive and equipped with rod, reel, and a few basic lures and see for yourself how many pointers you absorb in only one day. Devise and experiment with theories of your own too. In fishing, as in no other sport, you are the expert nearly from the beginning. Anything can work and the novel bait or technique often does. No other activity, besides gambling with cards and dice, takes "beginner's luck" as seriously. Fishing is a never-ending school where the fish always teach something new. Where the cocky angler is humbled by the wily, scaly creatures on a regular basis. Today's skunked (that means fishless) individual can be tomorrow's expert fisherperson. Truly, in fishing, you are never at the bottom—either emotionally or fish-wise—for long, if ever.

OVERCOMING PREJUDICES AGAINST FISHING

Many people, even those who do not fish, have definite opinions about the sport. "Fishing is for old men who have nothing better to do." "Kids can get a kick out of hooking a dumb fish but it is a waste of time for an adult." "Hanging your little bait in a body of water and hope for a fish to swallow it—Well, it's silly and one chance out of a million. Like looking for a needle in a haystack." These attitudes have one thing in common. They stem from childhood memories of how fishing was evaluated by mother and father—but especially father.

If the family was headed by an avid fisherman, he most likely headed for the stream alone or with a son who was perseverant, quiet, and had a temperamental affinity for angling. A daughter who is "Daddy's girl" may accompany him as a loving onlooker. But few girls are encouraged to fish. A number of mothers, ignorant of the rewards of fishing, pass on this prejudice against fishing to their daughters. In general, men exclude females, regardless of age, from angling, assuming they would be bored, restless, and inattentive. It is up to a woman to learn fishing on her own. Judge its spiritual and psychological benefits yourself. Pursue the type of fishing you like best alone or with a daughter or son. Do not permit custom to deprive you of a personally broadening, frustration-alleviating, self-satisfying outdoor activity. Find out for yourself whether fishing holds the same significance to your peace of mind that it does for 64 million anglers in the United States today.

SALTWATER FISHING

Saltwater fishing is angling for species of fish that live in salt water; in North America that means fishing in the Atlantic and Pacific oceans and the Gulf of Mexico. The fisher can set sights on a 2-pound mackerel, a 14-pound snook, or an 111-pound tarpon. The species of fish are nearly countless. Throw in a line to the turquoise liquid and wait for the mystery of what will take the bait. The time of year, water temperature, the presence of bait fish, and the tide work together to attract certain kinds of fish. The type of fish you will catch can be predicted, but within the vastness of the ocean there exists the possibility of surprise, the unusual.

Maybe you will hook a four-foot, snakelike needlefish or an evil-looking scorpionfish, besides the wahoo, yellowtail tuna, or the jack crevalle that were your primary targets.

The best place to learn about saltwater fishing is aboard a party boat. Aside from having a good time, the central activity is angling. A party boat consists of a group of fifteen to forty people who fish together for a day from the craft of a professional skipper. Anyone can reserve space on a party boat and catch fish. From New York City or San Francisco or Gulfport, Mississippi, sail with other anglers to the secret, sacred fishing grounds of the boat's captain. Fishing tackle can be rented and the novice can experiment with a variety of rods, reels, and lines until she finds one suited to her style. Bait is supplied on board.

Tell the deckhand that you are new at saltwater fishing and would appreciate suggestions. He will show you how to bait the hook. (Yes, to become a full-fledged fisher-woman, you must bait your own hook.) It is simple after the first couple of times. Remember, fish do not have human feelings. And the purpose of the existence of small fish, like anchovies and herring, is to be eaten by larger fish. Small fish are not necessarily young fish. Certain types of fish are called "bait fish," meaning they are the natural food of bigger fish.

Do not be too proud. The first time a fish nibbles the bait on the end of your line, you will experience a sensation akin to the pulse-quickening of your first love. When the line pulsates, jerk the rod upward with a quick movement of the wrists. This "sets the hook" and enables you to reel in the fish without losing it in the process.

Watch your comrades closely. Do what they do and ask questions. How deep to lower the bait and how to "drift" (or move) it are important factors in attracting fish. Observe closely those who are catching fish. Analyze what you are doing differently from them. Fishing looks simple. The angler with the most fish appears to be doing nothing except throwing the baited hook out into the water and then retrieving it with a jumping fish on the line. But, on the contrary, fishing is a sport of subtleties. The way the bait is threaded onto the hook gives it a natural and alive appearance. Where it is cast, how deep it sinks, and the speed of the retrieve play significant roles in catching fish.

On party boats, women can learn to fish with encouragement and assistance from companions, even though they may be strangers. A friendly atmosphere personifies the popular saying, "We're in the same boat, aren't we?" Even if she considers herself a "homebody," she can feel comfortable tackling this new sport of saltwater fishing aboard a craft that is run by the rule, "Everyone catches fish."

As added incentive to the party boat experience, each person usually donates a dollar to the "pot." The one who hauls in the biggest fish of the day wins the "jackpot." In this way, everyone is interested in the fish you catch. If it is a large one, it makes the other fishers on board try harder.

Meet Pat Snyder. She exemplifies in a true life way what each woman can accomplish in fishing if she wants to. Pat is primarily a wife and mother, living in California with her husband, Tom, and their two daughters, ages twenty-one and eighteen. During the first seven years of marriage, Pat conformed to society's norm for mothers. As she tells it:

While I stayed home and raised our two daughters, my husband went surf fishing on weekends and deep sea fishing on Wednesdays. This did it! I realized that I had to start joining him on these fishing trips or resign myself to being a "fish widow." I get seasick, but after bottles of Dramamine, learning to eat small amounts of food at frequent intervals, and some determination, this has become a very minor problem.

Believe it or not, I won the jackpot on the fishing trips the first three times we went out. This didn't settle too well with some of the old timers and veterans; especially since I didn't know how to hold the rod correctly. Talk about beginner's luck—but I was the one who was hooked!

Besides the thrill of the catch, I really discovered how relaxing it was to just be on the water—away from radio, telephones, TV and babies. My husband had always said it was the only way he had ever found to truly relax and I must say I echo his sentiments. Between the skipper, the mate, and a few helpful fishing buddies, I started my fishing career. That was about 15 years ago.

My husband used to attribute most of my fishing success to luck, but lately, even he has admitted I have developed and learned some skills. The secrets of proper reel drag and timing, for example, can never be taught to you. They are a matter of "feel."

The advice I offer to a woman who wants to fish is "Do it!" My oldest daughter loves to fish as much as I do and accompanies us on our trips whenever her schooling permits. She is good and will become even better with more time and experience. We encourage her to pursue her interest and hope someday she will have as much fun and time to fish as we have.

I have even gone fishing *without* my husband! In 1973, I had a rod custom-made for Tom for Father's Day. My enthusiasm for fishing frequently surpasses his and *he* was spending a day resting on the beach so our daughter, a girl friend of hers and I went fishing for the day (with me borrowing Tom's new rod).

I will never forget that day. I caught a 34 pound, 3 ounce roosterfish with that rod and a reel equipped with six-pound test line. [A six-pound test line means that the line breaks *under* six pounds of tension. If it breaks over six pounds, then it goes into the 12-pound category.] I registered it with the International Game Fishing Association (IGFA) and it is a world record. They call it a women's world record but my fish is also bigger than the current man's record roosterfish on six-pound line which is 29 pounds, 12 ounces.

I caught the roosterfish on six-pound Ande Tournament fishing line. The Ande Company used a picture of me with the record fish for their advertisement in the fishing and sports magazines nationwide. My ambition now is to return to Punta Colorada in Baja California in the next few months and try to better my own record. I'd love to have a 40-pounder.

While I was learning to fish, my husband stressed fishing etiquette. He is a hard fisherman but is extremely emphatic about proper ethics and manners when fishing. This was a good lesson to learn and has helped me when fishing with a boatload of men.

Fishing etiquette is really nothing more than good manners and having respect for your fellow fishermen as well as being honest and following the laws of nature and ecology.

1. When fishing on a boat with many others, *don't* allow your line to drift over another line.
2. When using live bait, watch your bait and know where it is at all times. Of course, this is not always possible because the bait swims wherever it wants to and you can't always see it. But try!
3. When another fisherman is "hooked up" (that is, he has hooked a fish), let him pass in front of you. Be alert for these things and don't wait to be asked or shoved! Let him follow his fish and bring your line in or keep it out of his way. The quickest way to "pop" a fish free is to cross lines.
4. The stern (rear) of the boat is usually the "choice" place to fish. When you have had your turn, rotate to the bow (front) or side rails to give everyone a fair chance.
5. Try to be an independent fisherman. Don't monopolize the time of the skipper, deckhand (or your husband) to bait your hook; take your fish off; unscramble your bird's nest (line tangled on the reel). A woman who fishes will gain added respect from the men aboard if she can handle her own problems and interfere with others as little as possible.
6. Learn to "hook" your own fish. Fishing is something you can't learn from a book. It's 90% "feel" as far as I'm concerned and the only way you can learn is to try it yourself and blow (lose) a few until you get the feel. I see too many women fishing who allow the deckhand or someone else hook the fish then all they do is crank it in. This is *not* fishing. My husband and I used to have arguments because he would want me to fight a fish he had hooked and I

refused. The "I'd rather do it myself" theory really holds true for me even if my fishing hasn't been good all day.

7. If a woman is to truly enjoy salt-water fishing, she must also learn to put up with a few inconveniences and discomforts. Bad weather, damp bunks (on a long fishing trip where you sleep aboard), cold, rain, dirty heads (toilets). I once looked around for the head on a 22-foot boat while fishing and could not find it. My husband finally located it *under* the seat cushion right next to the skipper (whom I'd never seen before in my life!) Try to solve that dilemma. A man has no problem at all with this inconvenience. But . . .

8. Listen to the advice of the captain on the boat. Some people go their merry way. But I find that the man who is in charge of the boat, who fishes for a living, knows more about the proper baits and methods than someone who goes out on a boat three or four times a year!

9. I *never* keep a fish unless I intend to eat it or give it to someone to eat. All the roosterfish I catch are released unless they are killed by the hook or unless I want to weigh a fish for a possible record. The same goes for all marlin and sailfish. I am honest and don't catch *over* the limit or keep any fish that is under-size. I want to have the fish around for many years to come so I can enjoy the sport with my husband and daughter. More than anything, I sure hope most other fishermen feel the same.

Let me also add I have found that fishermen (fisherpeople?) in general are wonderful, warm people. They are a special breed who all enjoy the sport, the outdoors, the fight of fishing; and respect others who enjoy it also. I love it so much.

Pat is one woman out of many who has adopted saltwater fishing as an expression of her love for life. Women who have no intention of pining away behind the walls of their homes, no matter how lovely. Now that they have reared

children and sacrificed for the betterment of their family,
they want to face the stimulation that the outdoors and
wild creatures incite. Mothers with young children can
begin now. Work pleasant activities like fishing into the
weekly schedule. Nature is waiting for you to finally discover her.

FRESHWATER FISHING

Freshwater fishing is the pursuit with rod, reel, and line of
fish inhabiting lakes, streams, rivers, ponds, and reservoirs.
Compared to the ocean, a lake is small with a very limited
array of life. But despite the physical dimensions, fresh
water affords pulsating sport. A lot of facts are known
about freshwater fish and for this reason catching can be
relatively predictable and frequent, even for the beginner.

Freshwater fish are classified into cold water and warm
water species. Trout—rainbow, cutthroat, golden, brown,
brook, dolly varden, and lake—live in cold water. So do
salmon and steelhead. These fish survive in water which
does not exceed 70°F during the summer. Found throughout the United States, populations of trout are concentrated
in the northern states. However, trout reside in deep lakes
and holes in the South also.

Bass, bluegill, sunfish, walleye, perch, catfish, and pike
are warm water species. Their environment can reach temperatures in the 90s without adverse effects on their systems.

Freshwater fish are usually smaller in size than most saltwater fish. A one-pound trout or half-pound bluegill is ideal
for dinner and can be a hardy contender for any angler.
Bass, catfish, walleyes, and pike live in lakes with relatively
long growing seasons. As a result, they can tip the scales
at eight to ten pounds. On light, freshwater tackle, tangling
with a fish that size is a sporty treat.

Find out at the local fish tackle or sporting goods store
or from a friend what type of fish is dominant in your area.
It makes a difference in the equipment you purchase and
the most effective baits to use. Before seeking instruction,
try fishing on your own, even if you do not know the first
thing about it. Until you attempt to cast the bait out into

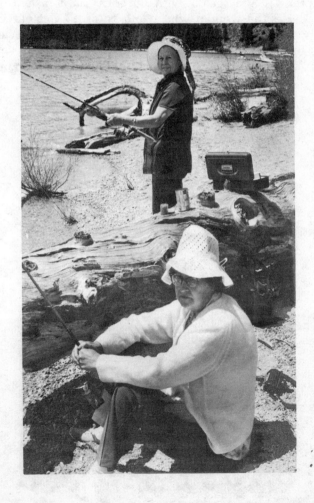

At Redfish Lake in Idaho, Elmira Scott and Ethel Bloomer fish for rainbow trout.

the stream, you will not understand why it is so important.

Borrow fishing equipment from a friend. Or purchase a rather inexpensive rod, reel, and selection of lures from your favorite discount house or sporting goods store. You are now ready for the challenge.

Joan Salvato Wulff's career revolves around fishing (see Chapter 1). She speaks with authority and insight when she advises the woman who wants to fish. "Get out there. The way to learn anything is to *do it*—over and over again . . . until a pattern develops and emerges. Observe and read . . . look, listen. Time spent alone in the outdoors can

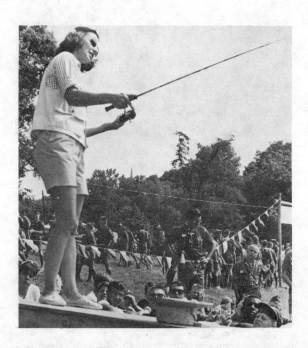

Joan Wulff encourages you to get out there and fish. It's fun.

make you a part of it and make you more sure of yourself in any natural setting. One of the first questions my husband (nationally known fishing authority, Lee Wulff) asked me when we met was, 'Do you go fishing alone?' Men have always gone into the outdoor world alone; women have tagged along, seemingly needing company. If we are to make our mark, we must do it alone, too, even if it is a *little harder* for us (and it is).

"I have observed that most men think women are a nuisance on a fishing trip, unless they are romantically involved with them. Because I have worked for tackle companies, since 1952, demonstrating their wares and giving clinics, I have been able to fish with top fishermen on an "equal" basis, without being romantically involved. They treat me with respect and yet are curious as to whether or not I will outperform them in the field."

Joan knows what she is talking about. Learn through an instructor or a friend but do not expect to break into fishing through your husband's guidance. Once you can call yourself a fisherwoman, he will undoubtedly be delighted and prefer to fish with you rather than with his buddies. However, the struggling, the frustration associated with the learning process, should be tolerated by you alone, with an instructor or within a class. Look forward to the first time you tie your own improved clinch knot that secures your own snap swivel to your line—which in turn fastens your lure. Wham! Your first fish. You have arrived. Welcome to the challenging, relaxing world of fishing.

Learn how to fish for trout and you can feel familiar with any other type of fishing.

Trout

A five-pound trout is big. Most trout run from one to two pounds. For the full fun of fishing, use a "light" rod and reel. The modern term is "ultralight." This means that the rod and reel together weigh only about nine ounces; this outfit transmits the battling of a one-pound trout to the angler. The rod is flexible. It doubles over under the weight

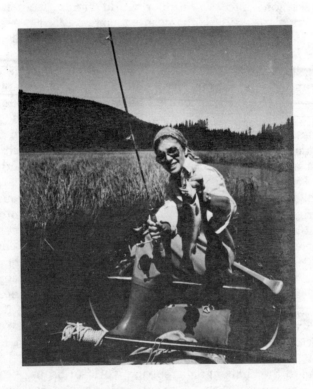

A 1½-pound brook trout was caught with this ultralight rod and open face reel.

of a four-pound fish. With an ultralight fishing outfit, playing (catching) a one-pound fish can be as exciting as hooking a thirty-pound saltwater fish. The ultralight rod and reel must have been designed with a woman in mind. You can hold the rod in the right hand and manipulate the reel handle with the left all day long without the arm or wrist feeling strain. In contrast, a bass rod and reel weigh approximately one pound, three ounces, about twice as heavy as an ultralight. The ten-ounce difference is noticeable and can produce aching muscles.

Casting. Spinning reels are either open face or closed face. The open face reel has no covering over the spool of line. Some say it is harder to cast than the closed face. But once you master casting with an open face reel, you can cast anything.

To cast the open face, first "flip the bail." The bail is a metal device on the reel, usually a chromed bar, that you flip on a spring to the opposite direction. Simultaneously, hold the fishing line in place with the top part of the index finger. Lift the rod tip up in the air and, with a little flick of the wrist, release the line from the index finger. The bait or lure will be propelled off the spool and land (hopefully) some distance away in the water. The next crank of the reel handle automatically snaps the bail back into the original position, which enables the caster to retrieve the line.

The closed face reel has a metal cover over the line. Advocates of this reel say the closed face reel does not have as many "birds' nests" as the open face version. However, if the line becomes tangled badly, the cover of the reel must be removed in order to unravel the mess. But this reel is easier to cast initially than the open face reel. Push the thumb lever on the reel all the way down. Release the lever at the full arc of the cast for a nice, smooth presentation.

Fly-fishing rod, reel, and line are completely different from spinning gear (see Chapter 1). Start with spin fish gear first. Experience the exhilaration of catching fish. Then, when you care more about testing your expertise than actually hooking and keeping fish, try fly-fishing.

At times, when fish are rising, dimpling the water surface in the evening and early morning, fly-fishing is a surefire method. The artificial fly can catch more fish than any other method because the fish are rising to and eating flies.

Fishing a fly is possible with spinning gear too by using the "bubble technique." A clear, plastic "bubble," available in tackle shops, is secured to the end of the line. Then, the fly, tied to a separate, foot-long piece of line, is fastened

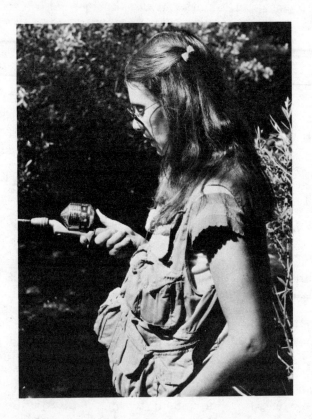

To cast a closed face spinning reel, push the thumb lever. At the full arc
of the cast, release the lever and the line will skim over the water surface.

to the main fishing line below the bubble. The bubble is
filled with water; this increases casting distance by giving
weight to the hollow float. The bubble still floats on top of
the water and suspends the fly behind it, retaining a natural
drift in the water.

Some streams and rivers are classified "fly-fishing only." In other words, only a fly can be used to attract and catch fish. This rule is common in many national parks, including Yellowstone Park. Within that park, the Madison, Firehole, and Gibbon rivers have fly-fishing only stretches. The bubble technique, using spin gear, is legal as well as the traditional fly-fishing method. To a novice, these regulations may sound confusing and unnecessary, but they demonstrate the responsibility of the fisher to learn the laws governing various bodies of water.

Baits, Lures, and Flies. Worms, dead minnows, soft cheese (like Velveeta brand), and miniature marshmallows are effective bait for trout. Bait is threaded onto a small hook. Hooks come in different sizes and are numbered accordingly. A number 0 hook, for instance, is big and a number 28 is minute. Between these extremes, the hook sizes vary with the larger numbers signifying smaller hooks.

Artificial baits are considered to be "higher class" in many fishing circles than real bait. Real or live bait is used when nothing else works. When the water is muddy, for example. In the minds of a number of anglers, using real bait is taking unfair advantage of the fish. However, bait fishing can be an art too—and the most enjoyable and relaxing type of fishing.

Artificials are divided into lures and flies. Lures come in all kinds of shapes, sizes, and colors. Spinners are lures with revolving blades that are designed to attract fish and help keep the spinner suspended in the water during the retrieve. Light in weight, they successfully lure trout. Fisherpeople in different parts of the country claim that the trout in their locale favor certain color combinations. For instance, red or orange-bladed spinners seem irresistible to brook trout in the Northwest. Determine what lure to use by asking other fishers and watching them closely. Persons who fish one area frequently have most likely pinpointed the favorite technique for catching fish. If all else fails, exercise imagination and come up with likely possibilities of your own.

A spoon is an oval-shaped piece of colored metal with a

treble (three-pronged) or single hook at one end. Spoons are usually heavier than spinners and sink quickly after being casted. Use a spoon where fish are lying deep, near the bottom of a hole. Small spoons work well on trout.

Trout, more than any other fish, have captivated the fantasies of humans. Frequently, while casting from a grassy bank into a gurgling stream, fishers have dreamed of being a trout. The kind of trout that is the focus of the aspiration depends on the individual's personality and what she considers important. Trout signify the wild, free spirit of the timbered North, where only the brave can weather the winter and love it.

Trout can be caught through the ice (of course, a hole is first drilled with an ice auger or chopped with a metal bar called a spud). For hungry wintertime fish, anglers will be forever grateful. While jiggling the bait or lure into the circular entrance to the frigid depths below, the fisher dreams of warm days and gentle breezes. Catching trout through the ice is an expression of hope for a summer to come soon and of better days ahead.

Trout appeal to the feelings that no one wants to discuss. They are an unspoken confirmation that the untamed part of city folk can be set free where concrete ends and the spongy layers of moss begin. Trout bring out the best in fishers and they love them for it.

Because the characteristics of trout endear themselves in the hearts of anglers, the question arises, "Aren't lures and baits with sharp, barbed hooks too harsh to use on our beloved trout?" And with that notion, fly-tying and fly-fishing came into being.

Lures are made of hard materials, like metal, wood, and plastic. But flies are hand-tied onto a small hook with thread, feathers, and animal hair. Flies are soft and closely resemble tiny aquatic or terrestrial insects that are natural food to fish.

The art of fly-tying has boomed within the past ten years. It is now big business, besides offering hours of solace from the daily routine. Fly-tying tides the fisher over during dreary winter months and muddy, rainy days. It primes fishing fever, but checks it from propagating into a full-blown plague. Fly-tying is an exacting, precise, detailed hobby that allows plenty of room for creativity. There is nothing in the world like catching a scrappy cutthroat trout on a Muddler Minnow, Renegade, or Montana nymph that you yourself tied.

Study Jack Dennis's *Western Trout Fly Tying Manual* (Snake River Books, 1974) for one of the most complete, step-by-step books on how to tie trout flies. *Basic Fly Fishing & Fly Tying* by Ray Ovington (Stackpole, 1973) covers fly-fishing for saltwater as well as freshwater fish.

Varieties of Trout. Devoted fisherpeople are inclined to attribute human qualities to trout, based on the distinctive habits of each kind. The brown trout, for instance, is a foreigner from Germany which emigrated to the United States in 1883. Stubborn and hard to catch, elder browns have a hooked jaw that seems to emphasize their wary nature. This trout survives relatively high water temperatures and silted waters where other trout would die. Bull-headed, ambitious, bold, and aggressive, Brownie relishes fresh fish (bait minnows, live or dead) for food.

On the other side of the coin lies the brook trout. Lovable and kind to anglers, she is nicknamed "Brookie." A native of the northeastern United States, she reproduces rapidly and strikes readily at the many offerings the fisher throws in her direction. Since the fish are prolific, even small brookies should be kept to prevent stunting from overpopulation. In short, the brook trout is an All-American fish, hitting anglers' bait democratically and rewarding them with a royal meal.

The cowgirl of the trout family is the cutthroat. Disclaiming her name (which would be more graphic of Ms. Brown trout), she is kind to strangers and likes to gulp the flies of eastern tourists who have traveled way out West to meet her. Quiet and shy, she cannot compete with the brown and rainbow and is usually replaced by them when they reside in the same water. She likes the wide open spaces and cannot bear the crowding and jostling of the browns and rainbows. Seldom exceeding five pounds, she is a small bundle of joy for any angler lucky enough to hook her.

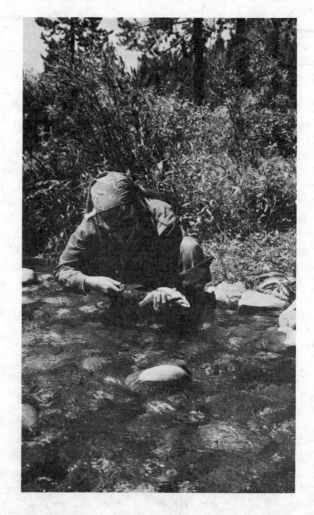

Here a brook trout is being cleaned.

What more can be said about lovely Dolly Varden? A spirited saloon gal, Dolly is native only to the Pacific slope. She is rather plentiful from British Columbia north, but has never really been transplanted to any great extent. Rough-and-tumble though, this char thrills western trouters. The Dolly Varden is called the glutton of the trout family and will eat anything from flies and insects to trout eggs and other fish.

The rainbow is a Pacific Coast transplant. Built like a heavyweight fighter, she doubles as an acrobat the moment she is hooked. With chilling leaps from the water and dancing on the surface, she stages a visual as well as a tactile display of her insistence on liberty. Restless, she likes to migrate and is more disease-resistant than other members of her family.

The lake trout is Ms. Big. Heavier and longer than her relatives, she also distinguishes herself by having a forked tail. Perhaps because of this unusual physical phenomenon, she cannot be trusted. With her needle-toothed mouth, she can easily slice a line and gain freedom. She feeds gluttonously on forage fish and is not the delicate eater that some of her cousins are. With an inclination for overindulging, she sometimes reaches obese proportions of sixty pounds.

In contrast to the eating habits of Ms. Lake are those of the golden trout. Small and delicate, she seldom achieves a weight of more than two pounds. She thrives in the thin air and short growing season of the cold, clean mountains of 10,000 feet or more elevation. Elusive and a selective eater, she prospers under severe conditions. She shuns civilization and offers sport only to rigorous backpackers who are willing to hike to reach her.

Within the trout group, there is variety and a fish personality for everyone's tastes. Trout are fun and challenging to woo because who can predict the behavior of such a temperamental family?

Bass

Bass are outstanding game fish and excellent to eat. Ferocious fighters, medium-weight tackle is required to catch them. Otherwise their tough mouths spit out the lure with hardly any effort. Since most bass run heavier than most trout, use a sturdy line of eight- to fifteen-pound test. Favorite foods of bass are minnows, crayfish (crawfish or crawdads), and worms.

Bass have conspicuously large mouths; in fact, one nickname for bass is "Bigmouth." More lures are designed and manufactured for bass than for any other fish. Plugs, spinners, spoons, floating and sinking minnows, deep divers, leadheads, rubber worms, and plastic poppers are just a few of the vast selection. Some fish theorists suggest that a bass attacks any foreign object that invades its territory. Aggression, rather than hunger, is the elementary bass motivator. Theoretically, you can attach whatever you want on the end of your line, cast it where the bass are sulking, and come up with a dynamite fish.

On hot days, bass will be lurking in deep water. For this reason, trolling is the preferred way of fishing. Once in bass waters, cast the artificial lure, real minnow, or other chosen bait behind the boat while it is moving at a speed fast enough to give the lure action in the water, but slow enough so the bait sinks deep. Let enough line out behind the boat so that the desired depth can be regulated. The more line you let out, the deeper your offering goes. With rod in hand, feel the bait working in the water. When a bass hits, give the rod a quick, powerful jerk upwards. Solid hook-setting is necessary because bass have thick lips and sinewy jaws.

Bluegill

Bluegill are flat-sided fish that usually grow no heavier than two pounds. Don't let their size fool you. This gamester has more spunk per ounce than any other fish. A respectable size bluegill is about as big as your hand with outstretched fingers.

Because bluegills are lightweights, use ultralight gear with tiny lures and flies. Easy to catch, most of the time—and delightful to eat—this fish has turned many a young girl or boy into a genuine fisherperson. Worms, crickets, or grubs are good bluegill baits. Cast the bait out and wait for the fish to swallow it. Reel in; put the fish in a creel (or on a stringer) and cast again. This process can be repeated many times during a day with the anticipation of a bluegill meal sparking you to catch more fish.

Little lures, like popping bugs with rubber legs or artificial flies (imitation red and black ants are good), attract bluegills. Because of a very small mouth, bluegill require minute baits and that's the key for catching them. If you feel fish hitting your offering, but cannot hook them, your bait is probably too large.

Catfish

Catfishing is a slow, relaxing type of angling. You can use just about anything for bait, from nightcrawlers to pungent doughball concoctions of your own formula. Throw your baited hook and line into a likely deep hole and wait. Meanwhile, chat or picnic. Play poker, read, or darn socks. Sitting at a catfish hole and soaking in the environment is the prime activity. Catching a catfish is a bonus.

Worms, dead minnows, or cut fish are reliable baits. You can create smelly doughballs and delicious (for catfish) blood baits. Even pieces of raw liver or chicken gizzard are prized baits. And catfish love entrails of any kind. The more repulsive and foul-smelling the bait, the faster catfish will engulf them with their large, wide mouths.

Because cats reach such a large size (especially blue cats and yellow cats), medium to heavy gear is generally recommended. For most types of catfish fishing, you can use your bass outfit.

Catfish could certainly fill the role as pets of Frankenstein. They are without a doubt, even to the most fervent lovers of God's creatures, grotesque-looking beasts. They have whiskers and can generally be described as black and slimy. But your affections for catfish will grow, the better you know them. After taking one or two off the hook, their looks will not be as abhorrent. Fishing for them can be fast and exciting. And they are, without a doubt, delicious eating. Deep-fried catfish fillets, fixed with corn fritters and hot, buttery biscuits, are hard to beat.

HOW TO TALK FISHING

Following is a glossary which translates the language of fishing for the beginner.

Angler's clippers: A pair of conventional fingernail clippers used by fisherpeople. They are handy for snipping monofilament line easily. Tie a pair to the fishing vest or carry in your pocket. After tying a snap swivel or lure onto the line, clip off the extra line to prevent spooking fish. Clippers can also be used to cut off lures and flies.

Bait-casting reel: A conventional, revolving spool fishing reel. Used primarily for bass fishing, ice fishing, and saltwater. As opposed to open and closed face spinning reels and fly-fishing reels.

Bait fish: Small fish, generally called minnows. Primary food of larger, predatory fish. Some saltwater bait fish include anchovies, herring, and sardines.

Bass: A warm water, freshwater fish, highly valued for fighting and eating qualities. Different varieties of bass are largemouth, smallmouth, spotted, and rock. There are also saltwater varieties including black sea bass, jewfish, and striped bass (found in both fresh and salt water).

Big game saltwater fish: Heavyweight fighters that can, and often do, weigh more than fifty pounds. They include tarpon, barracuda, marlin, sailfish, swordfish, tuna, and dolphin fish.

Bigmouth: A nickname for largemouth bass.

Bird's nest: An entanglement of the fishing line, consisting of many knots and inducing much frustration. Results from poor casts or retrieves or old, coiled fishing line.

Bite: Another name for strike or hit from a fish. A fish is biting when it mouths or nibbles the bait.

Bluegill: A hard-fighting freshwater sunfish and one of the most popular panfish. Called "bream" in the South. Average size is less than one-half pound.

Bobber: A plastic (usually red and white) ball-shaped device that floats on top of the water. It suspends bait off the bottom when it is positioned on the line at a desired depth. It also locates the bait. And the up-and-down bobbing movement denotes a nibbling fish. When it disappears beneath the water surface, the fish has swallowed the bait, signaling the fisher to set the hook.

Bobbin: Another name for bobber.

Bow (pronounced "bough"): The front or forward part of a boat or ship. As opposed to the back or stern.

Brook trout: A char moderately slender with minute scales. (Trout need *not* be scaled in preparation for eating.) Coloration is extremely variable but the front of the lower fins are usually lined white. Red spots dot the sides. Black blotches or dark olive bars commonly mark the back. Locally called "speckled trout" in some areas.

Brown trout: A fish with a brown or bronze hue and red spots on the sides. Old browns develop prominently hooked jaws. Browns are notoriously wary and often feed heavily at night.

Bubble: A clear, plastic sphere of bobbin size that can be filled with water. It is fastened to the fishing line and used as a float and to add casting weight. With the bubble, a fisher can cast even tiny dry flies without the use of a fly rod.

Casting: The process of presenting the bait, lure, or fly on the end of the line to fish in the water by means of a fishing rod and action of arm and wrist.

Catch-and-release: The fishing philosophy which promotes releasing any fish that is caught. Based on the premise that fish are a limited resource and that catching is more fun than keeping and eating.

Catfish: A scaleless fish with barbels (long feelers or whiskers) about the mouth. There are over 1,000 species of catfish in the world, including saltwater varieties. Most common in the United States are bullheads, channel cats, blue cats, and yellow cats.

Charter boat: A fishing craft that is hired with a skipper and mate for the exclusive use of one or a group of anglers.

Cleaning: Removing the entrails and scales from a fish with a knife to prepare it for cooking and eating.

Cork: Another name for bobber. A float to hold bait off the bottom and locate the hook. Made from cork, as opposed to plastic or wood.

Creel: A purselike container, with shoulder strap (and sometimes a harness), that keeps fish cool and prevents spoilage. Made of wicker or canvas and lined with freshly cut grass or permanent vinyl for easy washing. An angler carries either a creel or a stringer to retain fish.

Cutthroat trout: A cold water fish with black spots concentrated near the tail and red slash marks under the dentary bone, near the throat. The slashes or "cuts" on either side of the throat give the fish its obvious name.

Drag: A braking system on reels that produces an adjustable level of friction on the spool and line. The drag, a thin leather or Teflon diaphragm, allows the fisher to apply the desired pressure for the size and fight of the fish while reeling it in. A faulty drag is a major cause of lost fish, and one that is set too tight or too loose is responsible for the loss of many trophies.

Drift: Letting the bait, lure, or fly move with the current, tide, or wind. Not using the rod or reel to give the bait action, but letting it float naturally.

Eddy: A pocket of water near the bank, usually characterized by a slight reverse current. Most fish will rest and feed in eddies as opposed to feeding and resting in the main current. Eddies are best spots to cast to when float-fishing a river.

False casting: In fly-fishing, casting the line forward and backward without letting the line and fly fall on the water. This action is continued until the desired distance and line flow is reached. As the line is false casted, more line is fed into the rod guides; thus greater casting distances can be achieved.

Filleting: A way of preparing fish for cooking in which the slab of meat on each side of the fish's backbone is cut away. Two boneless fillets result from one fish, leaving head, tail, back, and rib cage as waste.

Fishing etiquette: The unspoken manners, consideration, and respect each fisher should extend to her companions, the fish, and the environment.

Fishing vest: A sleeveless jacket with many small pockets which hold tiny boxes of fishing lures, flies, and other gear. Some vests feature built-in mesh creels where fish can be stored as soon as they are caught. Vests are, in reality, portable tackle boxes and are handy when walking and fishing the banks of a stream or lake.

Flipping the bail: On an open face spinning reel, moving the bail (a metal, chromed bar that operates on a spring mechanism) in the opposite direction. This frees the fishing line and permits casting. After the cast, the first crank of the reel handle automatically snaps the bail in the original position. The bail then rewinds the line onto the spool of the reel when the handle is turned.

Float: Another name for bobber. Or to "float" a stream when fishing.

Fly-fishing: The art and science that deals with catching fish by means of an artificial fly that is tied to imitate a natural insect. The fly rod is used to make a natural presentation of the fly so it lands softly on the water. The fly is actually cast by the weight of the fly line, rather than the fly reel, which is merely a line-storage device. The basic fly cast is a graceful unrolling of the line by false casting and the delicate placement of the fly where fish are suspected to be.

Fly reel: A revolving spool with a small handle that is attached near the butt of the fly rod. To cast, the fly-fisher strips line from the reel and works the rod and line back and forth as in false casting. The fly reel is not directly involved with the process of casting like a spinning or baitcasting reel.

Fly-tying: The art of creating artificial insects that resemble the aquatic and terrestrial foods that fish eat. The main ingredients, besides the hook, are animal hair, rooster feathers ("hackle"), and thread.

Golden trout: A relatively small, slender fish, bright golden yellow below the lateral line and with black spots in the tail and dorsal fins. Found in mountain lakes usually above 10,000 feet in elevation.

Grayling: A freshwater fish that inhabits cold, clear lakes and streams of the North. The fish is not common by U.S. standards. It is identified by a prominent dorsal (top) fin and brilliant colors ranging from gray-green to blue-silver. It is a highly prized game and eating fish.

Hit: A strike or bite.

Hole: A relatively deep pool of water in a stream, river, or lake where fish are likely to congregate for rest, food, or escape from periods of extreme heat or cold. Holes are the prime places to fish.

Hooks: Curved pieces of steel wire with barbs used for catching and holding fish. Hook sizes vary according to the size, mouth, and toughness of the sought-after fish. A trout needs a small hook, while a bass requires a larger one. Hooks come in different sizes and are numbered accordingly. A number 0 hook is large, while a number 28 is minute.

Hookup: The situation that exists when an angler has a fish on her line and is trying to bring it in. According to etiquette, she has the "right of way" on a boat or stream. Other fishers should move away from the hookup or reel in their lines.

Ice auger: A hand- or gas-powered corkscrew or drill-bit device that bores holes through the thick or thin ice for the purpose of ice fishing.

IGFA: International Game Fish Association, 3000 East Las Olas Boulevard, Fort Lauderdale, Florida 33316. A center for the exchange of information on marine angling grounds, seasons, fishes, and record catches.

Improved clinch knot: The knot used for attaching hook, fly, or swivel to the fishing line. It involves wrapping the loose end around the line four or five times, then slipping the end through the resulting loop and again back through the loop to prevent slipping. A good, all-around knot to use.

Jackpot: Each angler on a party boat donates a specified amount of money (usually one dollar) to the "pot." The person who catches the largest fish of the day wins all the money in the jackpot. The winner usually tips the skipper and mate with a portion of the winnings.

Jigging: A method of fishing in which the angler lowers the lure or bait to the desired depth and imparts movement to it by jerking the wrist and rod upward and then letting the lure or bait flutter downward. Especially effective for ice fishing or crappie fishing in fresh water and deadly on some

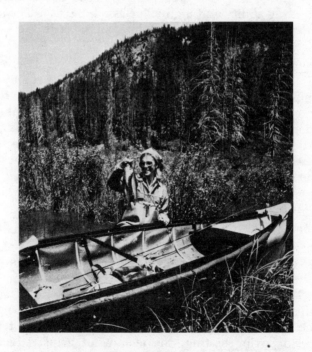

A stringer of keepers entitles the fisher to a little boasting.

bottom-feeding saltwater species. Most "jigs" have lead heads and tails of feather or Maribou.

Keeper: A fish of respectable size that promises good eating, along with sufficient boasting or bragging.

Lake trout: A char with a forked tail and gray blotches against a dark body. Also known in some areas as Mackinaw.

Landing a fish: The action involved in retrieving a fish from water. Fish, when played long enough, wear down. Reel in, keeping the rod tip up and line taut. This helps control the fish's movements. When the fish is close, secure it with a landing net; slide it on the bank, or reach down and grab the fish behind the gills with thumb and forefinger. Remember, some fish have extremely sharp fins or teeth and can seriously cut when not handled properly.

Largemouth: A type of bass that is pursued for its outstanding fighting ability and high value as a table fish. The largemouth is one of the most popular game fish in the United States.

Leader: In fly-fishing, commonly a nine- or twelve-foot length of fine, monofilament line that connects the fly with the main fly line. The leader is supposed to be nearly invisible to fish and gives a natural appearance to the fly. Leaders are sold in varying tapers, lengths, thicknesses, and breaking strains. The size of a leader is measured in tippet size, which is the diameter and breaking strain of the smallest part of the leader. In spin fishing, a leader may be a two-foot length of monofilament line that is attached to the heavier main line.

Leeward: The direction toward which the wind blows. Opposed to windward.

Level-wind: On bait-casting reels, a chromed wire guide that travels back and forth on a rotating track built into the reel. The line is threaded through the guide and is laid on the turning spool in uniform layers. When casting, the guide directs the line off the reel. When the proper thumb tension is added during casting, the level-wind helps reduce the chances of "backlash" or birds' nests caused by the line bunching up and tangling.

Limit: The number of fish that the state game and fish department or the federal Fish and Wildlife Service dictates that an angler can catch and keep from a specific body of water. Catching more than the limit is illegal and subject to prosecution. In some states, there are both number and weight limits on sport fish.

Line weight: In fly-fishing, the amount of pressure a fly line can tolerate, measured in grains and based on the first thirty feet of line. The weight of line should be coordinated with the weight and length of the fly rod. And it should be sufficient to work the rod so that it produces a graceful, smooth curling and unrolling of the line during forward and backward casting movements. A number 6 fly line weighs 160 grains and can tolerate pressure from 152 to 168 grains. Lower numbers refer to lighter lines while higher numbers designate heavier lines. Number 6 is average, number 3 is light, and number 12 is heavy.

Lunker: A large fish, usually a trophy of a species.

Medium-weight gear: A relatively stout fishing rod with eight- to twelve-pound test line and suitable reel with the capacity to handle that line. A typical bass spinning or bait-casting fishing outfit would be medium-weight gear as compared to ultralight or heavy, off-shore fishing equipment.

Monofilament: A popular type of nylon fishing line made from resin that comes in a variety of colors and is rated by its breaking strength. Twenty years ago most lines were cotton, dacron, or braided nylon that often became saturated with water and difficult to cast.

Mouthing the bait: Instead of immediately consuming the fisher's offering, the fish investigates it first, with its mouth. A bumping or tugging sensation warns the angler to wait a few seconds before setting the hook. Otherwise, the fish will feel the barb and flee, wiser to the ways of fishers. Largemouth bass, for instance, will often mouth a plastic worm or eel before swallowing it.

Nibble: What fish sometimes do to bait. An announcement to the angler to set the hook.

Panfish: Any fresh- or saltwater fish that can be fried whole in an average-size frypan. Commonly applied, however, to bluegill, sunfish, perch, or crappie.

Party boat: A group of fishermen who fish for a fee from a craft, or party boat, of a professional skipper.

Perch (yellow): A panfish that provides excellent eating. A member of the pike family and characterized by yellow-gold color and six to eight broad, vertical, black bars that extend from the back nearly to the belly.

Pike: Large freshwater fish that have gained a reputation as ferocious fighters. Pike have cannibalistic eating habits and favor large minnows as food. These fish have elongated bodies and prominent snouts filled with razorsharp teeth. Bean-shaped, light-colored markings speckle the sides. The fins are usually spotted with darker blotches.

Playing a fish: Reeling in the fish carefully and steadily with rod tip up and line fairly taut. Give the fish its head when it dives deep or swims off in another direction. The fish works against the drag of the reel. When it tires, reel in to recover line. Do not try to "muscle" or "horse" the fish into the boat or shore. Increased tension on the line might break it and the fish would be lost.

Pliers: A pair of pliers, especially the point-nosed variety used for fishing, is a convenient tool for the angler. Use pliers to remove the hook from the mouth of a fish. Most fish have teeth of some kind and pliers prevent the hands from being scratched. They can also be used for clamping split shot onto the line and for general tackle repair.

Plug: A lure made of plastic or wood that wobbles or swims when the fisherperson supplies the action through rod and line. Some plugs float while others sink just under the water surface or deeper. Plugs come in a variety of shapes and colors to imitate bait minnows or fish. They are especially effective for bass (both fresh- and saltwater) and pike.

Pole: A "folksy" name for a fishing rod. A cane or wooden pole was the first fishing rod, and such poles are still used by many anglers today.

Pool: A large hole where placid, deep water attracts fish to rest and feed. A good place to fish on a stream or river.

Pop the line: After the fish is hooked, the line breaks, freeing the fish. This can be caused by friction of the taut line against submerged rocks or against the side of the boat. Fins and sharp teeth can also "pop" the line.

Popper: A plug created mainly to resemble a frog, injured fish, or insect on top of the water. It is retrieved in short jerks. A popper can have a tail of feathers, hair or rubber skirt, and rubber legs. Poppers are used effectively for bass and bluegill fishing.

Popular saltwater fish: Bluefish, bonefish, bonito, croaker, cobia, dolphin, flounder, grouper, mackerel, mullet, perch, striped bass, pompano, sheepshead, snapper, snook, tarpon, tuna, wahoo, and weakfish.

Pound test: A manufacturer's measurement of fishing line that describes the pounds of tension a line can tolerate before it breaks. A four-pound test line, for example, should break under four pounds of tension. The trick of catching large fish on a light line is to play the fish until it tires. The angler uses the give-and-take of the long rod to wear down the fish. This type of fishing demands skill and patience. While playing the fish, the angler must not exert so much force that the line breaks. Yet she should not allow undue slack in the line which could enable the fish to spit out the hook.

Rainbow trout: Normally deeper in body than the cutthroat trout, it has a smaller mouth. In addition, black spots cover the body, head, and fins. No red spots. A broad band, ranging from orange to pink or red, sweeps the body laterally; thus the name "rainbow."

Retrieve: Reeling in the lure or bait. Retrieve varies from slow to fast and smooth to jerky. Various types of retrieve are used for different fishing conditions and species of fish. When and where to employ different types of retrieves is an important key to fishing success.

Riffle: A rocky and relatively shallow section of the stream, where the water jumps over rocks. Either above or below a riffle usually can be found a hole where fish congregate to feed. These are especially good spots to fish.

Rise: An increasing circle or dimple on the water surface signifies a rise. A fish rises to gulp an insect from the water surface. This usually means a hatch of insects has descended on the stream or has emerged from the bottom of the stream or lake and that fly-fishing would be the most effective method. A rise pinpoints where a fish is lying, waiting for food. Cast the fly so it drifts through the circle of the rise.

Rod: For most fishing conditions, a fiberglass shaft anywhere from six to eight feet long that is tapered from butt to tip and equipped with line guides. The rod supports a fishing reel and line and with it an angler can cast, set the hook, and retrieve a fish.

Salmon: A game and food fish with silver scales. Some species of salmon live in saltwater and spawn in fresh water. Others are landlocked in lakes and rivers. Some of the popular salmons are chinook, king, atlantic, and coho.

Setting the Hook: A quick, upward jerk of the wrist when a tugging or strike is felt on the other end of the line.

Sinker: A lead weight attached to the fishing line. The added weight enables the bait or lure to sink into deep holes where fish are. Sinkers also aid in long-range casting. They come in different shapes and sizes. There are rubber core sinkers, slip sinkers, trolling sinkers, bell sinkers, and split shot.

Skunked: Going home fishless.

Spawn: Fish eggs. Or the process of fish laying their eggs.

Spinner: A lure with thin blades that rotate when retrieved through the water. Spinners come in a variety of colors and weights. They are especially effective for trout.

Spinning reel: A stationary spool fishing reel that enables line to coil off the spool as a result of the casting motion of the angler. As opposed to the revolving spool bait-casting reel. Spinning reels are either open or closed face.

Split shot: A tiny sinker made of lead shot, with a slit in one side that enables the shot to be clamped onto the fishing line with a pair of point-nosed pliers. Split shot comes in different sizes and is numbered accordingly. Shot is good for stream fishing in order to get bait or fly down deeper in the

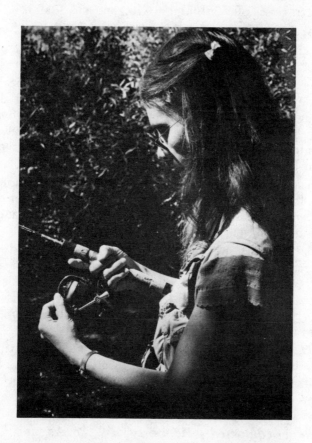

This is how to flip the bail on an open face spinning reel.

current. Split shot can be added or subtracted to reach the desired fishing depth.

Spoon: An oval-shaped piece of colored metal with a treble or single hook at one end. This lure wobbles through the water when retrieved. It sinks fast and is made to resemble a fleeing minnow or bait fish.

Starboard: The righthand side of a boat or ship as one faces forward, towards the bow. As opposed to port.

Steelhead: A sea-run, rainbow trout that is common in western rivers of Washington, Oregon, and Idaho.

Stern: Rear of a boat or ship. As opposed to bow.

Strike: A fish hitting or grabbing a lure. The fisher responds by setting the hook.

Stringer: A metal chain with large, safety-pin type holding devices. Undo one of the safety pin clips and slip it through the lips or gill and mouth of the fish. Fasten the safety pin. Tie the stringer to a stick, rock, or boat. The restrained fish is then put in the water to be kept alive and fresh. Most stringers hold about ten fish.

Sunfish: Small freshwater fish, including bluegill, pumpkinseed, bream, shellcrackers. Easily caught on worms or grasshoppers, sunfish are a delight to catch for young and old alike on light gear.

Swivel: Made of metal, it consists of a tiny, barrel body with a wire loop at either end or a wire loop at one end and a tiny, safety-pin type attaching device on the other. A swivel or snap swivel joins the fishing line to the lure. It also prevents twisting of the lure that could entangle the fishing line. A swivel adds to the ease of changing lures.

Tackle box: A portable container, made of plastic, metal, or wood, that holds most fishing gear, except rods. It organizes fishing equipment into one box and helps the fisher know what gear she has and where she can find it. Most boxes have compartmented trays that hold lures.

Terminal equipment: Hooks, swivels, sinkers, and fishing "hardware" in general.

Timing: Setting the hook at the right moment so as not to spook the fish and miss it.

Tippet: In fly-fishing, the smallest diameter of the leader to which the fly or hook is tied. It can be very fine, almost hairlike in diameter, and is about two feet long. It allows the artificial fly to drift and float naturally in the current.

Troll: To fish from a moving boat which is used to carry bait or lure into the water. Speed of the boat determines how deep the bait can be fished. And the more line let out, the deeper the bait. Trolling is a good technique for locating schools of fish.

Ultralight: Very lightweight spinning gear ideal for fishing trout and panfish. Rod and reel together weigh about nine ounces. With such lightweight gear a sporting fight and pull of the fish is transmitted through the line and rod. Even catching small fish can be fun.

Undersize fish: A fish too small to eat or under legal size. That is, usually less than six inches long. As opposed to a keeper.

Waders: Rubber, waterproof boots that come in hip or chest lengths. Useful for stream fishers who need to wade out into the water to reach a particular hole. Waders fit over the clothes and socks. Shoes are removed before putting them on.

Walleye: A member of the pike family with large mouth and sharp teeth. The fish gets its name from the large, bulging, opaque (glassy) eyes. A popular sport fish, generally with a dark olive green back and lighter sides, mottled with yellow. The walleye is considered to be among the finest eating of the freshwater fishes.

12

Hunting

Artie thought she was special. And not many contradicted her. She had been shooting arrows from a bow since she could walk. At age seven, she could hit the bull's-eye of the buckskin target when she concentrated extra hard. She shoved everything from her mind except the silver dollar-size black spot. She imagined that dot was really in her eye. She was looking through the bull's-eye, with the bull's-eye and at it all at the same time. The target was part of her. An important part. Maybe even vital. Her mind carried her there, about fifty yards away, and it must have directed the arrow as well. Because she rarely missed.

Lay a vase on its side fifty paces away with the neck facing Artie. She could shoot an arrow into it. She thought that an oak-shafted arrow with tanager feathers was as pretty as a flower. It belonged in a handmade, sun-baked, pottery vase. Beauty, speed, accuracy, and power all rolled into one.

The bow and arrow were not primarily weapons to Artie. They were means of self-expression. Her twin brother Pollo liked to tease her. His favorite nickname for her was Beanstalk because her physique resembled one—tall and skinny. To ease the hurt, she reached for the bow and arrow and calmly, deliberately punctured one knothole after another on the wooden fence surrounding home. After awhile, bad feelings left and she could smile again. No one could deny she was the best archer in the county.

The graceful, elegant bow contains more strength within its curved construction than the archer could ever hope to have. It is perfect for a woman. Especially, one like Artie who craved precision and was not afraid to work for it. While friends disappointed, angered, and disillusioned her at times, the trusty bow was consistent and stable. It always felt the same in her hands. Smooth and dependable. But beneath that exterior lurked a tough core, an unbeatable spirit, and deadly accuracy. Artie had a lot in common with the bow.

Artie's real name is Artemis. Her brother is Apollo and their father is Zeus. She was one of the twelve great Olympian Greek deities who lived thousands of years ago, at least in the minds of those who prayed and offered sacrifices to her. She was the goddess of hunting, archery, and a defender of wild animals, children, and weak creatures. She brought fertility to women, as well as death. And she protected newborns.

Apollo, her twin, was the god of music and medicine. Like Artemis, he was held responsible for the sudden but natural death of men.

In short, Artemis and Apollo were the mythological explanations for the apparent incongruities of existence. For instance, they were the reasons why some beings were weak while others were strong. Why a few were sterile. Why all living creatures must die. These Olympian twins were invented to help humans understand the incomprehensible, the injustices of life. But the influence of Artemis and Apollo went beyond the human realm. They also regulated the numbers of game animals and the quantity of food in the pantries of the townsfolk. The abundance of herbs, the amount of leisure time, the creation of beautiful music and the splendid things of life were under the direction of Artemis and Apollo.

The Greeks and other primitive people created goddesses of hunting. Even though males commonly were the hunters, they turned to mythical females for direction and guidance. Why? Because the female represented fertility. Even though the hunters wanted to kill game, their primary consideration was to have an ample supply of wild animals for the future. Hunters slew animals to feed their families. But they wisely realized that game was a limited resource and needed replenishing. A goddess could ensure this because she too knew the value of reproduction, of continuing the species. For early communities, the existence of wild animals guaranteed a reprieve from hunger and starvation. Without game to hunt, kill, and eat, humans would perish.

IRRATIONAL ATTITUDES AGAINST HUNTING

Nowadays, the word hunting is likely to trigger a heated, emotional debate, especially in metropolitan areas far removed from the wilderness where game abounds. Many people imagine the wilds as a giant zoo where innocent, stupid animals wait around for hunters to appear and shoot them. The current theme of antihunting is becoming a popular issue to which people donate time, energy, and money. It is based, however, on misconceptions about the nature and needs of wild animals, the fear of guns, and the mystery of death.

In the first place, hunting does not necessarily mean killing. An outdoor photographer can "hunt" animals and birds with the camera. Wildlife photography involves many of the preliminaries that hunting with a gun does: locating an animal's territory, identifying its habits and carefully pursuing it until "shooting" range is reached. But the photographer pushes the shutter button instead of pulling a trigger. The advantage of hunting with a camera is that you can enjoy the excitement of the stalk and the adventure of creeping within fifty yards of the animal any time of the year. You do not have to wait until hunting season, when animals are more suspicious, wary, and less likely to allow humans to get close.

In a similar way, a woodswoman can hunt wild flowers, mushrooms, songbirds, edible plants, valuable rocks and fossils, or other treasures that only the outdoors can offer. To discover what you have been searching for can be a thrilling, rewarding experience. However, it cannot match an actual hunt where you meet an animal on its own ground for a life-and-death struggle.

Traditionally, "hunting" describes a person using a rifle or shotgun to pursue an animal or bird. To many city dwellers, the idea of using a gun is the offensive part of hunting. A majority of suburbanites have grown up with the false impression that a gun represents crime or lawlessness. Unless as a young girl she has had experience with a BB gun or a .22 rifle, a woman probably fears guns and what they are capable of doing.

Actually, a gun is a safe instrument. It is more difficult to accidentally injure yourself or another person with a gun than it is with a knife. Every gun is equipped with a safety lock that, when functioning as it should, makes it impossible to fire a rifle. With proper knowledge of gun handling, slip-ups are rare. Each hunter treats her gun with the utmost respect. When you fully realize the power and force of a rifle, the more cautious and careful you become. It is ignorance of guns, and the correct way to handle them, that causes problems. Accidents are likely to happen among unknowing children or to people who have not had proper gun safety instruction.

GUN SAFETY INSTRUCTION

Courses on gun safety and handling are offered by local chapters of the National Rifle Association (NRA). Some local trap and skeet shooting clubs also offer sound courses for all age groups. And fish and game departments throughout the country now incorporate in-person or televised classes into their programs. Hunter safety classes are most often advertised in advance of hunting season over radio or television or in the outdoor pages of the local newspaper.

The best way to overcome an irrational fear of guns is to learn about them and actually handle them. Fire at a safe

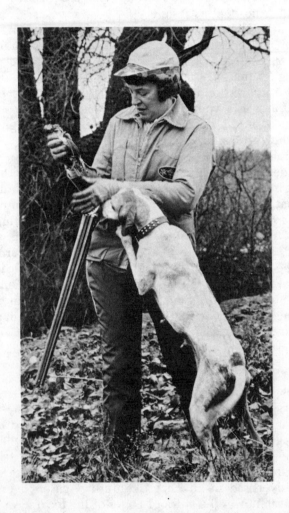

Joan Cone is a Hunter Safety Instructor. Here she puts a quail which she has shot with a shotgun in her game bag.—*Photo by John Avery*

target and experience for yourself how a rifle feels and what it can do. A gun is merely an extension of the person using it and most people are capable shooters. Society trusts the vast majority of automobile drivers. Yet cars are potentially more destructive than guns. The key to good gun safety and handling is education. Shooters should attend safety and handling courses which require that a certificate of expertise be earned before taking the field.

THE AMERICAN TRADITION OF HUNTING

Hunting is much more than firing a gun or an arrow at a wild animal. A tradition that extends back to the beginning of the human race, hunting insured the survival and prosperity of your ancestors. In fact, it is the only fundamental activity that ties modern with prehistoric humans. Basically, hunting is the only history that the United States has. Besides the Constitution, it is the only legacy handed down to today's outdoorspeople by their forebears.

WILD GAME MEAT AS A MONEYSAVER

To a hunter, killing an animal or bird is not absolutely vital to enjoying the sport or feeding the family. However, a freezer full of wild game meat reduces the grocery bill considerably. An average-size mule deer buck, for instance, weighs about 200 pounds. Mature antelope weigh in the neighborhood of 110 pounds, and a bull elk will tip the scales around 600. One antelope, one deer, and one elk can feed a family of four during a year's time.

In terms of beef, two 1,000-pound steers would feed that same family for an equivalent number of months. There is more fat and waste on beef.

TODAY'S ODDS FOR HUNTING SUCCESS

Hunting means getting out into nature and directing your wits and energies towards fooling an animal or bird on its own ground. This is not easy. Animals are amazingly smart. National hunter success is most often only 50 percent or lower. In 1974, for example, more than ten million Americans purchased licenses to hunt deer, the most popular of the big game hunting species. Approximately two million deer were harvested. The hunter success percentage was about 20 percent. Only one out of every five hunters actually shot a deer. Considering the accuracy and high quality of today's firearms, this low success ratio is a significant tribute to the instinctive intelligence and guile of deer. The number of deer harvested is in no way threatening the population of the national deer herd. In fact, most deer numbers are quite a bit higher than they were fifty years ago. Selective harvesting of game animals is a tool which modern game managers use to balance a certain number of animals to the carrying capacity of available habitat. The most serious threat to game animals today is loss of habitat.

The bowhunting harvest is only about 3 percent of the gun harvest. In 1974, Pennsylvania bowhunters harvested 3,880 deer while New York archers killed 3,206 animals. Compare these figures with the 2,600 deer that were slaughtered by cars on Pennsylvania highways in 1974. Bowhunting provides a lot of sport for a lot of hunters without significantly reducing game herds.

Hunting in the United States today is always a challenge. There is nothing really sure or predictable about success. At least a day-long hike is required in most hunting situations. There are tracks to discover and follow and animal signs to decode. And there is a good chance you will walk a lot of miles without even firing the rifle.

Even if you spot an animal, getting within shooting range is quite a different matter. Some nimrods talk about "high-powered rifles." A 30.06 (pronounced thirty-ought-six) or a 7mm Magnum has the capability of killing an animal quickly and surely within 400 yards, which is a long distance. However, through a scope on the rifle, an antelope at that distance looks like a dot—no bigger than the tip of your little finger. To kill the animal at that distance takes a lot of luck and a great deal of knowledge about your rifle. In other words, it is a long shot, literally and figuratively.

An antelope can run fast—sometimes in bursts to sixty miles per hour. In a matter of minutes, it can be miles away

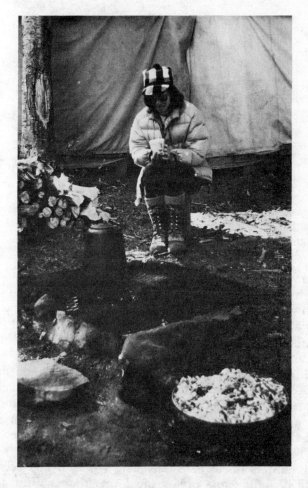

Hunting is much more than firing a gun or an arrow at a wild animal. It is a tradition and a complete, quality outdoor experience.

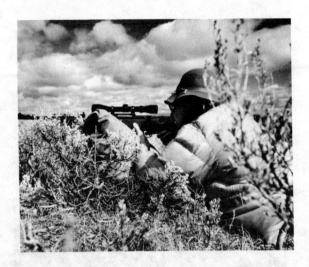

A high-powered rifle, like this 30.06, is used for hunting western big game, like antelope, deer, elk, moose, bighorn sheep, and mountain goat and bear.

from you. Hunting is a matter of outwitting an animal that is much better equipped to meet the challenges of the terrain than you are. Sometimes luck turns the table. That is when the hunter gets an opportunity for a shot. But before thoughts can turn to venison steaks, a good shot has to be made. This takes skill and practice.

Hunting is one of the toughest challenges for modern woodswomen. It is much more difficult than parachuting from a plane or skiing a steep slope or driving a stock car. You are dueling with a wild creature. The best animal wins, and the odds today are definitely in favor of the beast.

Through hunting, a person develops a respect for animals that borders on awe. Rarely can a person appreciate the guile of wild game unless she hunts them. Wild animals are not meant to be pets or to be caged behind bars in a zoo. They are not "cute" or "funny." They are independent.

Humans are infringing on their existence, however, by taking over their habitat. The frantic search for precious minerals, oil, and coal and the resultant destruction of habitat is much more dangerous to wildlife than hunting is. Whereas hunting motivates animals to sharpen innate skills, the loss of habitat leaves them at the mercy of the elements. They are forced into smaller quarters; disease often spreads and the entire herd can be wiped out.

In many areas, domestic cattle and sheep graze heavily on public Forest Service and BLM lands during the summer. Consequently, there is less food for wildlife during the winter when they desperately need it. Where ranchers spray and kill sagebrush to cultivate public land with hay for cattle, antelope and sage grouse as well as rabbits, badgers, hawks, eagles, and songbirds have less food and shelter. These animals and birds depend on natural forage for existence. Without it, they die.

The independence of wild game makes them particularly attractive to hunters. For those who have not had experience with wild game, it is hard to believe that animals survive without human patronage. Antihunters feel that wildlife should be protected and preserved whether they need it or not. These people are against the sport of hunting and do not want hunters to hunt. They are organizing movements to take away the right to hunt. Through lobby groups in Washington, D.C., they are trying to impose their own norms, based on misunderstanding, on outdoorspeople.

THE BAMBI COMPLEX

The false belief that animals are cute, gentle, and humanlike and need protection and care from humans, characterizes the Bambi complex. Today's young adults grew up with Bambi, a deer in an animated cartoon by Walt Disney. Granted Disney gave the American public a great deal in terms of family entertainment. But, he also did a disservice to people and animals alike by humanizing wild creatures. In his stories, animals have a social structure and family life much like humans. In the end, they want to serve and be pets of humans. His characters are at peace with each other and nature and live in perfect harmony. Disney portrayed a perpetual Garden of Eden. A lovely idea and beautiful picture but simply not a realistic representation of the animal world.

Nothing in nature is static. Everything eventually suffers and dies, including humans. The life-and-death struggle among animals occurs dramatically, and sometimes brutally, each day. Before modern conveniences were invented, humans likewise participated in the fight for survival as they do in poor countries today. But Americans are far removed from these stark realities and want to push them from consciousness. They wish to ignore the fact that they are creatures too. That they are not the centers of the universe or the world. By believing that people and wildlife can live in a Disney-type peace, humans seek happiness without pain. The anti-hunting movement, then, is really a misplaced expression of despair over the current state of human affairs.

HOW HUNTING HELPS WILDLIFE SURVIVAL

In truth, modern-day hunting is based on sound biological principles. A certain percentage of animals should be harvested each year from the herd to keep the rest of the animals strong and healthy. Hunting prevents wild creatures from becoming diluted and tame. Without hunting, overpopulation would trigger overgrazing, lack of food, and eventual starvation.

This is exactly what happened at Great Swamp National Wildlife Refuge in northern New Jersey. From 1970 to 1974, an estimated forty whitetail deer died there of starvation or diseases associated with the stress of overpopulation. Wildlife biologists warned that unless limited hunting was allowed on the refuge, the entire herd would collapse.

On December 10, 1974, a U.S. district court in New Jersey gave the order permitting hunting at the refuge. Biological data received showed that 127 deer were harvested by 638 hunters over 6 days of hunting. About half of the harvested deer were closely examined by game biologists. According to the studies, 45 percent of the deer were

infected with an organism that causes peritonitis. Lung-
worms were found in 12.5 percent. Body weight was four-
teen pounds lighter than the average New Jersey deer. In
22 percent of the whitetails, veterinarians discovered tape-
worm larvae, that normally contaminate the livers of dogs
and cats. Never before had tapeworms been found in deer.

Poor nutrition, from overpopulation and lack of food,
weakened the normally immune system of the deer. As a
result, diseases that a healthy deer could fight off would
probably have been fatal to deer in the overpopulated herd.
One refuge buck, for example, was covered by tumors,
called Papillomatosis, which is caused by a virus. While
a healthy deer might have one or two tiny nodules the size
of BBs, this particular buck was blinded by the rampant
development of huge growths over his entire body.

Hunting on the refuge was sanctioned by the court as a
humane way of limiting the deer population and to save
the animals from a slow, pitiful death from starvation or
other unnatural afflictions.

In the past, hunting and killing game for food was a
necessity. Our specialized society, with modern agricultural
practices and efficient food distribution, has taken the hunting out of killing for food. Instead masses of domestic animals are killed in slaughterhouses. The animals are bred
and raised and fattened in pens just for this purpose, to die
as food for Americans. Is this more acceptable to the social
conscience than hunting? Is killing on a production-line
basis more desirable than participating in the hunting
tradition that has helped perpetuate today's wildlife herds?

The Bambi complex has insidiously permeated people's
attitudes towards animals. Animals appear to be beautiful,
magnificent, naive, and vulnerable. Especially those wild
animals that have inhabited preserves where hunting is not
allowed. They seem almost tame. But occasionally a Yellowstone black bear mauls a potato-chip feeding tourist who
ventures too close. Or a sedate, apparently heedless buffalo
suddenly wheels and gores the photographer that dares to
venture within inches.

Wild animals, even ones protected from hunters, cannot
be truly domesticated. They protect themselves through

violent means when they feel threatened. If not hunted, approximately 10 to 20 percent of a wildlife herd will die of old age, disease, starvation, predators, exposure, and highway loss annually. Whether you want to admit it or not, each living organism must die. Blame it on Goddess Artemis, hunters, or overpopulation, but the fact remains and no amount of legislation against firearms and hunting will change that.

LEARNING HOW TO HUNT

Hunting is much more than firing a rifle at an animal or aiming a shotgun at a bird. It is a complicated process in which a human engages in a battle of wits with an animal. Hunting can take a lifetime to learn. Yet even experienced hunters have difficulty predicting and fooling game animals and birds. Besides the mechanics of shooting, hunting is mostly intuition. It is asking yourself, "If I were a deer, where would I be on a beautiful, fall, sunshiny day like today?" Hunting is a philosophy that instructs its followers, never give up. At the moment you are least prepared, a deer will walk within yards of you. Experience, too, that helpless situation when you have placed your shotgun on the ground and are in the process of crawling through a barbed wire fence. Pheasants then explode from hideouts all around you. Or take the times when you are settling down to a midday sandwich, a thermos of hot chocolate, and a doze. As if someone turned on a switch, squirrels begin chattering in every direction even though they were silent and invisible all morning.

Hunting can be an emotional, meaningful experience. One that can hold a special place in your thoughts for the rest of your life. Of all the outdoor activities, hunting hits closest to the central core of what being an outdoor person is all about. It rekindles the primitive human in each person and helps bridge the centuries between then and now.

Suzy Sherer could be a twentieth-century Artemis. No one offers her sacrifices or prays to her for guidance and plentiful game. But throughout her home state of Idaho, she is recognized as an outstanding huntress. She and her husband Ron recently built a home in Eagle, not far from Boise, where Ron serves as a fireman. They and their two children, fourteen-year-old Susie and twelve-year-old Mike, live on a ten-acre minifarm with six dogs (used for tracking game), two horses, one steer, and one pig.

Besides being wife and mother, Suzy was the first woman to shoot a Rocky Mountain bighorn sheep and a Rocky Mountain goat in Idaho. She also successfully hunted a black bear with a bow and arrow. "Locating the bear was not hard as we (my husband and I) knew there were some in this specific area. We set off to the hills with four of our hound dogs. Our strike dog found a fresh set of tracks and took off running. At one point, the bear ran right past my husband. He had to jump off the path to let the bear run by. After about an hour chase, the bear finally treed. I was frightened as I had never seen a bear this close before. He hissed, snarled, popped his teeth and growled. I would shoot an arrow and then run behind another tree . . . then back to the spot again to shoot another arrow. My hits were good and he came down out of the tree and hit hard. He weighed about 150 pounds, an average size bear. Even though he was brown in color, he is classed as a Black Bear."

Suzy used a forty-seven-pound bow, which means the bow required a pull of forty-seven pounds to draw it to the fullest. For a woman to shoot such a bow accurately, daily practice at drawing and aiming is required. Suzy developed the necessary strength over a period of twelve years of archery, both in the field hunting and in target competition with women of the same class of shooting skill.

But the hours of physical exertion paid off for her. "Archery has given me a sense of accomplishment. I have never been a very forward person. My years of archery have made me a better person with more confidence. I worked for many years to be number one. The hardest part was staying there and trying to accept new challengers. I have received many trophies of various shapes and designs, which I dust off regularly with a nice feeling of appreciation. However, they are not the reasons I continue with the sport. They are just the happy results."

By stopping a black bear with a bow and arrow, Suzy was entitled to join the Pope and Young Club. This is an elite organization of outstanding archers, mostly men, who have bagged trophy big game using bow and arrow. There are about 1,000 members throughout the country who have qualified themselves as members. Of these, only about thirty are women. Suzy Sherer is one of them.

"In hunting, I take my chances just like the next 'guy.' I neither expect or receive any favoritism. I have climbed many mountains just for one shot at a deer, but that is a fulfillment in itself. When I shot my Bighorn Sheep, I cried right after I shot it. I guess this was just releasing my tension and unraveling my pentup nerves. I had laid on a canyon rim for over two hours just watching the sheep, waiting for the right opportunity and hoping they would not spot us. This was frustrating as I felt this was my one, big, chance—to do something no other woman in Idaho had done—to shoot a bighorn ram.

"My advice to women who want to become knowledgeable about archery and hunting would be to get professional assistance on archery. Clubs, for instance, give correct shooting techniques in classes. A thorough knowledge of archery is needed before you can ever expect to go hunting. Know the terrain, conditions and the type of game within your hunting area. Scout the area beforehand. Dress according to the weather conditions.

"I feel lucky to have had the opportunities and the exposure I have had. I am truly satisfied that I have probably seen more variety of game and been through more hunting conditions than most men will ever see in their lifetimes. This is my satisfaction. I feel my husband respects me for being able to enjoy the sport as much as he does. He encourages me in archery. He tries to convince me not just to compete with others, but to try and do what I think I am capable of doing. This has helped my attitude toward archery. Trying to shoot for myself and not be psyched out by competitors.

"We have tried to encourage both our children to know the art of hunting and to enjoy the sport. Both shoot archery. My daughter Susie is a good huntress. She shot her first game last fall. It was an antelope shot with my trusty .243 rifle.

"Some men have told me they wish their wives were like me and really enjoyed hunting and the outdoors. To me, this is a compliment and it makes me feel like I am not just the ordinary housewife or working mother."

Besides desire, hunting requires steady nerves, physical coordination, and good eyesight. The eye can be trained to spot game, especially when binoculars are employed in "glassing" a game area. Good hunters wear their binoculars almost constantly and spend a lot of time carefully glassing the hills for signs of movement or color that is out of place. If you can hold your own in a tennis match, putt a golf ball with some degree of accuracy, or pick off a single pin when bowling, you have the eye-hand coordination of a huntress. But the finer points of hunting can be learned only by doing.

An avid hunter who is also a friend may be willing to teach you. Or you can contact a hunting guide who advertises in outdoor magazines. Female guides are few and far between at present. So you will probably have to choose a man who has a good degree of patience. A guide that specializes in small game hunting for rabbits or birds would be a good choice. You will then have plenty of opportunities for shots and have the thrill of hunting with beagles or bird dogs that make hunting even more fun.

Trained hunting dogs—beagles and German short-haired pointers, for instance—prepare you for the sudden appearance of game. When beagles bay or pointers brace and point, shoulder your shotgun and wait for rabbits, quail, or pheasants to burst from cover. Even then, quickness is the difference between going home emptyhanded, tired, and frustrated or enjoying the main course under glass at home later.

Marlene Simons, a professional hunting guide (see Chapter 3), is also a National Rifle Association instructor. She understands the problems that the novice huntress faces and has groomed many into excellent markswomen. In addition, she is willing to educate women on the finer points of big game hunting. Unfortunately, most of her hunters are men. She would like to see more women participating in the sport of hunting. She counsels, "If you plan on taking up hunting with a rifle or shotgun, get into a good NRA class and learn everything you can about your rifle. How to handle it and shoot it safely. This is a big gripe with men who complain that most women are careless handlers of guns."

BEST GUNS TO USE

To test your reaction to guns, begin with a .22 rifle. It is a relatively small, compact firearm that is easy to hold steady. The recoil (the rearward motion caused by the force that propels the bullet out of the barrel) is slight. In fact, by holding the rifle firmly against the shoulder, the recoil is hardly noticeable. The report, or noise, caused by firing the .22 rifle is similar to that of a cap gun.

Practice squeezing the trigger. Aim at a variety of safe targets such as aluminum cans, the joker from a deck of cards, or the bull's-eye of a standard paper target. Predict where the bullet will hit. Fire, and see how close to the mark you are. Shoot the .22 from a number of positions—that is, sitting, standing, or prone (on the stomach).

In most states, squirrels and rabbits can be hunted using a .22 rifle. One cartridge at a time is fired. And because the .22 is a rather small cartridge, accuracy is paramount. If you can shoot a rabbit in the head with a .22 cartridge, you are ready to hunt any type of game.

Bird and small game hunters usually carry shotguns and most shotgunners prefer the 12-gauge. A shotgun is a smoothbore gun that fires a charge of lead shot. It expels the charge from a plastic or waxed cardboard hull, in patterns that vary from tight (full choke) to wide (improved cylinder) like the nozzle of a hose. The middle pattern range is called modified. A shotgunner has a choice of bore patterns when choosing a single-barreled gun. A side-by-side double barrel or over-under barrels usually have two bores in one gun. A general rule of thumb to follow is choosing improved cylinder for shooting at birds under thirty yards and modified or full for ducks or geese over thirty yards.

Accuracy with a shotgun is less a matter of aiming than

it is pointing. Unlike the single projectile of a rifle's bullet, the shotgun emits tiny, lead pellets (shot) that can be diverted into impotency by heavy wind or brush. Shotgunning demands a great deal of practice, especially at moving targets such as clay pigeons. With enough practice, eventually shotgunning becomes second nature and the gun feels like a third arm.

In certain states in the East, shotguns are the only legal type of hunting guns. Rifles are outlawed. But in the West, high-powered big game rifles are widely used. Rifles are classified according to caliber (the diameter of the bore of a rifle before the rifling grooves are cut, measured in hundredths of inches —.20, .30, etc.). The .22 rifle is ideal for learning but the .30 calibers are suited for big game hunting. The .30-30 and the .30-06 are western favorites. However, a .243 can be effective for big game hunting. The key to clean, fast kills is the placement of the bullet in the heart or lungs of the animal. Good hunters strive for accuracy and consistency of bullet placement.

The recoil and report of a shotgun and big game rifle are considerable when compared to the .22. Big game rifles can be hand-held, but accuracy suffers. A rest, such as a tree limb or boulder, steadies the rifle and ensures good bullet placement. When practicing with a big game rifle, wear ear plugs to blot out the noise and a thick jacket or vest to cushion the shoulder. Ironically, when firing at elk or moose, or any game animal for that matter, the awareness of recoil and report is negligible. Adrenalin makes the difference. The shotgun does not warrant this amount of protection. Practice will accustom the hunter to the noise and punch of the shotgun.

For women, the 20-gauge shotgun is light and easy to handle. It has less recoil than the 12-gauge, that is favored by male scattergunners. Hunters who use a 20-gauge swear it equals a 12-gauge in performance. The key to consistent shotgunning is aiming at targets that are within the 40-yard range. That's when pellet density is at its best, and the chances of a clean kill are most favorable.

Unlike a rifle, a shotgun is rarely equipped with a shoulder sling and is carried ready to shoot at all times. This position can put considerable strain on the forearms towards the end of a day of walking through cattails, briar patches, and heavy underbrush. The shotgun often feels more like a cannon. For this reason, it is best to choose the lightest gun possible and one that feels right in your arms and shoulders. Many times, women try to fit themselves to their guns, whereas shooting accuracy depends on the gun fitting you properly from the start. Basically, this means that the distance from gunstock butt to trigger approximates the distance from elbow joint to the second joint of the index finger. A gunsmith can alter the gunstock to fit your shooting reach. For the shotgun to become part of you, it has to fit the size of your body.

OVERCOMING MALE PREJUDICE

Learning about guns is only the first step. Next comes the practical experience. As Marlene Simons explains, "In the field of hunting, there are so many articles written about what duds we women are that all men get the same impression. . . . If women want to change men's attitudes about women hunters then they themselves will have to do it. Be knowledgeable about your sport. . . . Read everything you can. Then if you do go hunting with your favorite guy, be sure not to complain. If you are well read you should know what you are getting into."

Women also tend to give a poor impression about their hunting savvy, Marlene points out, "when they start talking about the poor, big-eyed animal that will be shot and how they hate to cook the game meat. Properly cooking wild game is a really good place to start."

When you realize how good game meat is, you will have an added incentive to hunt.

"One article I read in *Sports Afield* talked about this hunter who went into the woods opening day and found his favorite stump occupied by a woman. The writer went on to say that women had no place hunting. I wrote him a letter inviting him on a hunting trip but he wouldn't take me up on it. A real authority!"

Joyce MacDuffie of Helena, Montana agrees with Marlene and goes one step further. "I believe that women have been discriminated against in the outdoor field. . . . It is fine for women to write on how to cook an elk steak but *never* on how to hunt an elk; kill an elk; or butcher one in the field. I had the dubious distinction of being the only female in the U.S. or Canada to ever head up a state hunter safety program. At the time I was running Montana's program, there were 30 states and six Canadian provinces which had statewide hunter safety programs and the other 35 were run by men. Now there are programs in all 50 states and in eight Canadian provinces and all 58 are run by men. (Not making much progress are we?)"

Joan Cone (see Chapter 1) is a Hunter Safety Instructor for the NRA. At age thirty, she learned to hunt with her husband and after seventeen years of hunting experience— "We get out at least once weekly from October until March" —she has several firsthand tips for women who would like to hunt. "Many men confide in me that they wish their own wives or girl friends would join them outdoors. A good many men get fed up going out with 'Good ol' Charley' and would prefer to be with someone whose company they enjoy more. Men's main objections to women in many cases, is about those who whine and complain about conditions like rain, wind or other hardships."

Sheila Link (see Chapter 1) is a spirited huntress who has successfully pursued deer, bear, elk, wild turkey, mountain sheep, upland game, and waterfowl. She was featured on "The American Sportsman" show on ABC-TV on February 18, 1973. The cameras followed and recorded her bighorn sheep hunt, which took place in British Columbia. She shot a respectable ram with one cartridge at a distance of about 100 yards. And the television viewing audience was there watching her expressions and hearing her reactions.

She sums up the role of women in hunting. "There is a certain amount of so-called 'discrimination' shown outdoor women. This is not, in my opinion, however, a conscious effort to frustrate us. It stems, instead, from a paucity of sincere, enthusiastic outdoorswomen. In hunting camps, for example, separate bunkrooms are not common—because women hunters (unless accompanied by a husband) are uncommon.

"A good choice of outdoor clothing, boots and scaled-to-size equipment is unavailable too, simply because manufacturers have learned that there's not a big enough market to warrant production on any but a limited scale. If changes are to take place, I think it will be up to sportswomen to force them. Not by mere demands, but by becoming numerous and visible enough to encourage change."

There is the challenge. The rewards are found wherever you turn in nature. But the entire cycle of the outdoor experience must begin in your heart where you are someone special—a doer, a woodswoman. Continue the tradition from the goddess Artemis—to you.

Bibliography

Angier, Bradford. *Living Off the Country*. Harrisburg, Pa.: Stackpole Co., 1956.

Bauer, Erwin A. *Hunting with a Camera*. New York: Winchester Press, 1974.

———. *Outdoor Photography*. New York: Times Mirror, Book Publishing Division, 1974.

Bauer, Erwin, and Bauer, Peggy (eds.). *Camper's Digest*. Second Edition. Chicago: Follett Publishing Co., 1974.

Blaisdell, Harold F. *The Philosophical Fisherman*. Boston: Houghton Mifflin Co., 1969.

Borror, Donald J., and White, Richard E. *A Field Guide to Insects of America North of Mexico*. Boston: Houghton Mifflin Co., 1970.

Camera, The. *Life* Library of Photography. New York: Time, Inc., 1970.

Cannon, Ray. *The Sea of Cortez*. Menlo Park, Calif.: Lane Magazine & Book Co., 1966.

Carroll, Jon. "The Electric Gatorade Superstar Test." *womenSports*, Vol. 2, No. 4, April, 1975, pp. 36-42.

Comstock, Anna Botsford. *Handbook of Nature-Study.* Twenty-fourth Edition. Ithaca, N.Y.: Comstock Publishing Assoc., 1960.

Dennis, Jack H., Jr. *Western Trout Fly Tying Manual.* Jackson, Wyo.: Snake River Books, 1974.

Disley, John. *Orienteering.* A Rubicon paperback. Harrisburg, Pa.: Stackpole Co., 1973.

East, Ben. *The Ben East Hunting Book. Popular Science/ Outdoor Life* Book. New York: Harper & Row, 1974.

Farmer, Charles J. *Creative Fishing.* Harrisburg, Pa.: Stackpole Co., 1973.

Farmer, Charles, and Farmer, Kathy (eds.). *Campground Cooking.* Northfield, Ill.: Digest Books, 1974.

Findley, Rowe, and Edwards, Walter Meayers. *Great American Deserts.* Washington, D.C.: National Geographic Society, 1972.

Frazier, Neta Lohnes. *Sacajawea, The Girl Nobody Knows.* New York: David McKay Co., 1967.

Fritzen, D. K. *The Rock Hunter's Field Manual.* New York: Harper & Brothers, 1959.

Gabrielson, Ira N. (ed.). *The New Fisherman's Encyclopedia.* Second Edition. Harrisburg, Pa.: Stackpole Co., 1964.

Gillelan, G. Howard. *Modern ABC's of Bow & Arrow.* Harrisburg, Pa.: Stackpole Co., 1967.

Gipe, George. "Yesterday." *Sports Illustrated,* Vol. 42, No. 13, March 31, 1975, p. W4.

Grant, Michael, and Hazel, John. *Gods and Mortals in Classical Mythology.* Springfield, Mass.: G. & C. Merriam Co., 1973.

Green, Jim. *Fly Casting from the Beginning.* California: Fenwick/Sevenstrand, 1971.

Grimal, Pierre (ed.). *Larousse World Mythology.* New York: G. P. Putnam's Sons, 1963.

Harbour, Dave, and Harbour, Bobbie. "1975 Sports Afield Deer Survey and Hunt Planning Guide." *Sports Afield,* Vol. 173, No. 6, June, 1975, pp. 66-74.

Hebard, Grace Raymond. *Sacajawea.* California: Arthur H. Clark Co., 1933.

Hidy, Vernon S., and editors of *Sports Illustrated. Fly Fishing.* Philadelphia: J. B. Lippincott Co., 1972.

Johnson, Cy. *Western Gem Hunters Atlas.* Susanville, Calif.: Cy Johnson, 1969.

Kelly, Fanny. *My Captivity Among the Sioux Indians.* New York: Corinth Books, 1962.

King, Billie Jean, with Chapin, Kim. *Billie Jean.* New York: Harper & Row, 1974.

Kjellstrom, Bjorn. *Be Expert with Map and Compass.* Stackpole Co., 1967.

Knight, Doug. "Insect Repellents: which ones work and why." "The vitamin that keeps bugs away." "All about those pretty green plants that give you fits." *Sports Afield,* Vol. 174, No. 1, July, 1975, pp. 40-43, 44, and 46-47, respectively.

Latham, Sid. *Camera Afield.* Harrisburg, Pa.: Stackpole Co., 1976.

Light and Film. Life Library of Photography. New York: Time, Inc., 1972.

McDonald, Elvin. *The World Book of House Plants.* New York: World Publishing Co., 1963.

Milne, Lorus, and Milne, Margery. *The Nature of Animals.* Philadelphia: J. B. Lippincott Co., 1969.

"Ms. Dreidame Looks for Golden Age." *Alumnus* (University of Dayton), February, 1975, p. 27.

Mohney, Russ. *The Master Backpacker.* Harrisburg, Pa.: Stackpole Co., 1976.

NRA Staff. "The Great Swamp Hunt." *The American Hunter,* Vol. 3, No. 5, May, 1975, pp. 18-21.

O'Connor, Jack. *Complete Book of Rifles and Shotguns.* Second Edition. New York: Harper & Row, 1965.

O'Connor, Jack. *Complete Book of Shooting.* New York: Harper & Row, 1965.

Ormond, Clyde. *Complete Book of Outdoor Lore.* New York: Harper & Row, 1964.

Ovington, Ray. *Basic Fly Fishing & Fly Tying.* Harrisburg, Pa.: Stackpole Co., 1973.

Photographing Nature. Life Library of Photography. New York: Time, Inc., 1971.

Pilley, Dorothy. *Climbing Days.* London: Martin Secker & Warburg Ltd., 1965.

Powell, J. W. *The Exploration of the Colorado River and Its Canyons.* New York: Dover Publications, 1961.

Robbins, Chandler S.; Bruun, Bertel; Zim, Herbert S.; and Singer, Arthur. *Birds of North America.* Wisconsin: Western Publishing Co., 1966.

Search for Solitude. Washington, D.C.: U.S. Dept. of Agriculture, Forest Service, 1970.

Simon, James R. *Wyoming Fishes.* Bulletin No. 4. Revised Edition. Cheyenne, Wyo.: Wyoming Game and Fish Department, 1951.

Sosin, Mark (ed.). *Angler's Bible.* South Hackensack, N.J.: Stoeger Publishing Co., 1975.

Telander, Rick. "A voice for those long silent." *Sports Illustrated,* Vol. 42, No. 26, June 30, 1975, pp. 60-63.

Webster's New World Dictionary of the American Language. College Edition. New York: World Publishing Co., 1962.

Wyoming Collecting Localities. Wheatland, Wyo.: Eloxite Corp., 1965.

Wyoming Rockhunter's Guide. Cheyenne, Wyo.: Cheyenne Mineral and Gem Society, 1965.

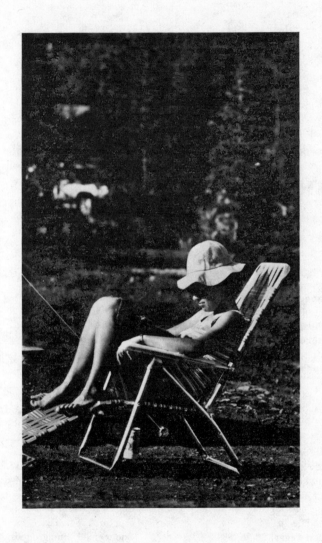

Index